THE FIVE TIBETANS BREATHING BOOK

A Guide to Deeper, Slower, and Easier Breathing
With The Five Tibetan Rites – Boosts Longevity,
Vitality and Health

Other Works by Carolinda Witt

The Illustrated Five Tibetan Rites
The Eye of Revelation 1939 & 1946 Editions Combined
Double Agent Celery MI5's Crooked Hero
The 10-Minute Rejuvenation Plan

THE
FIVE TIBETANS
BREATHING
BOOK

A Guide to Deeper, Slower, and Easier Breathing With The Five Tibetan Rites – Boosts Longevity, Vitality and Health

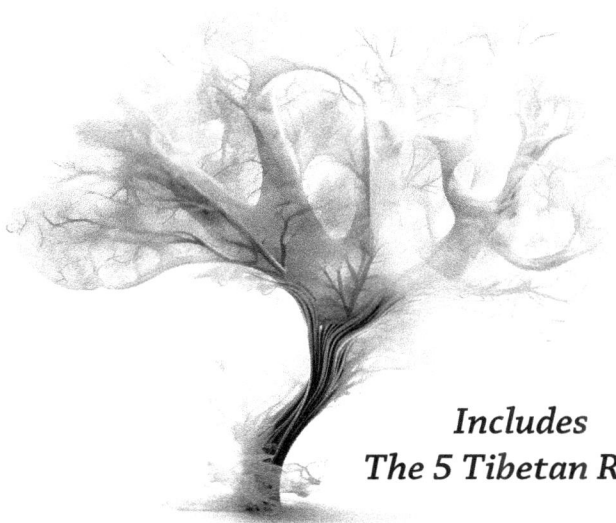

*Includes
The 5 Tibetan Rites*

CAROLINDA WITT

THE FIVE TIBETANS BREATHING BOOK

**A Guide To Deeper, Slower, And Easier Breathing With
The Five Tibetan Rites – Boosts Longevity, Vitality And Health.**

Paperback ISBN: 978-0-9870703-5-7
eBook ISBN: 978-0-9870703-9-5

UnMind Pty Ltd
PO Box 818, NSW 2107, Australia

Visit the author's website at www.T5T.com
T5T is a registered trademark.

Photographs, 2005 by Steven Murray
Cover Design: Damonza
Interior Design: Lazar Kackarovski

A catalogue record for this book is available from the National Library of Australia

Year of publication: 2024

To Holly, Joss, Tess, Archer, and Benji, witnessing your earliest breaths was one of the greatest miracles of my life.

TESTIMONIALS

My chiropractor recommended that I learn T5T to improve my health. I used to experience a feeling that I couldn't breathe before learning the Energy Breathing method in T5T. The very first moment I started practicing it, I felt that I could at last draw a full breath. This was a very rewarding experience for me. Being involved in the health industry has enabled me to seek out many alternatives to improve my health and well-being, but none have been as profound as practicing T5T daily. The health benefits for me personally have been enormous: increased flexibility, stronger neck, back, and abdominals, huge improvements in my breathing patterns, and increased mental clarity and focus. I believe T5T is the perfect complement to any healthcare system that people may have already chosen.

—**Lynda Santich,**
Natural Health Industry Entrepreneur

Breathing slower, deeper, and easier is vital for longevity, health, and vitality. I believe that T5T can help most people become more conscious of their breathing. It can also release tension in their breathing, and often gradually expand their breathing capacity as well as slow their breathing rate.

—**Michael Grant White,**
"The Breathing Coach," Optimal Breathing Academy

I work as an Airline pilot and am finding the benefits from both core muscle development and breathing exercises.

—Brian Fogerty, Airline Pilot

I breathe better than I ever have, and through that, I have improved my relationship with my family, which includes a calmness I'd not really experienced before. I cannot recommend this program highly enough, and as it only takes me ten minutes a day, it is hardly a sacrifice of my time.

—Robyn Gilbey, Publicist

I find that I have more focus, and I don't freak out when I have school exams and stuff, and I'd like to say that the breathing, I think, is very beneficial.

—Rose Ricketson, (age 15), Australia

I like the daily focus on breathing - the explanations in the book are really informative and clear. As a breathing coach, I know how incredibly important it is to breathe correctly, and Carolinda's method will certainly help most people breathe deeper, slower, and fuller.

—Jan Jenson, OBDS
(Optimal Breathing Specialist) from NC, USA

I also find the breathing to be energizing and rejuvenating, allowing me to embrace challenges and function at an optimal level.

—Jillian Naidu, Sign Language (Deaf) Interpreter

The silent migraines I have been experiencing for years have almost disappeared, and my energy levels have increased tremendously (I used to have days that were so bad I could do nothing but sit and sleep in a recliner chair all day). I wake up feeling rested, breathing is better (likely due to all of the controlled breathing that the exercises require), and almost no coughing, sinus pain, and headaches gone, and very little post nasal drip (again likely due to the controlled nasal breathing), far less grumpy (that happens to some of us older guys), less cold, digestion much improved and much, much more. I just notice that as each week passes I am feeling better and better. The only change I have made in my life has been adding the T5T exercises.

—Robert Wilkie, Canada

I never thought it would be possible to gain more energy and become more relaxed in only 10 minutes a day. But T5T manages just that. Amazing.

—Paul Wilson,
Bestselling author of *"The Little Book Of Calm"*

I have practiced yoga for many years, but after having a baby (my third child), I needed some exercise that would put me back in shape and that took as little time as possible to do! T5T has been exactly what I needed. Now, if I miss a day or two, I feel unbalanced, uncentred, and have low energy. They are so simple yet so powerful in their effect.

—Susan Hayward,
Bestselling author of *"A Guide To The Advanced Soul"*

As an osteopath, I was looking for an exercise routine that incorporated mind, body, and spirit - something that was going to give me energy, strength, and flexibility. I spend a lot of time bending over a bench and need good core stability to support my lower back, and T5T has given me this. As an osteopath, I see many people injure themselves doing exercise they are not in condition for. However, what I like about T5T is that it is a gradual step by step program, taught safely and under close supervision. This enables gradual strength, flexibility, and core stability to develop - thereby minimizing the risk of injury. The breathing and relaxation techniques complement the rites and provide a solid platform for increased body and mind connection. These benefits, combined with ancient wisdom, make T5T a powerful daily ritual, and I recommend it to all my patients and anyone who wants improved health and vitality.

—**Libby Ross, Registered Osteopath**

For me, the whole system, including the energy breathing, really feels like it's having a big impact on my internal health. Now, T5T is the first thing I do every day. That says it all.

—**Richard Meikle, Master Personal Trainer**

ACKNOWLEDGMENTS

I am grateful for the support and knowledge of breathing expert and coach Michael Grant White, who has shared so much with me over many years—and for writing the foreword of this book. My breathwork and meditation teachers who guided my interest in mindfulness and energy-raising breathing techniques, including Holotropic Breathing, Kriya Yoga (SRF), Prānāyāma, Yoga, and the Art of Living Foundation's *Sudarshan Kriya*. Author and teacher Dennis Lewis for his profound insights into the consciousness-raising aspects of breathing and its relationship to inner growth and health, and Donna Farhi, yoga and breathing instructor, for her knowledge and clarity in describing the natural movement of the breath. Over the years, many health practitioners and experts have shared insights and advice, in particular, physiotherapist and yoga teacher Susie Lapin and osteopath Dr. Libby Ross for their full-hearted support and guidance in helping me develop the step-by-step method of learning The Five Tibetan Rites, which I call T5T. Julie Gibbs, publishing director of Lantern/Penguin books, for publishing my first book on The Five Tibetan Rites and making it look so beautiful.

TABLE OF CONTENTS

FOREWORD

As a long-term yoga and health practitioner, Carolinda had undertaken training in specialized breathing techniques and was mystified by the absence of breathing with The Five Tibetan Rites.

When I met Carolinda over twenty years ago, she was finalizing the material for her The Five Tibetan Rites workshops, blending ancient practices with modern knowledge. She booked several private sessions with me, outlining her aim to create a daily wellness routine that blended natural, full breathing with the Rites. Carolinda explained her principal focus was on teaching people how to experience the movement of their breathing muscles and spaces of the body—and then apply that learning to establishing better breathing practices—fuller, slower, and easier. The goal behind her approach was that, through daily repetition of these principles and practices, people would become more aware of when their breathing was suboptimal in everyday situations—and be able to adjust it accordingly.

Irregular breathing patterns affect how we feel, think, sleep, and move and are far more common than people realize—we all do them. Stress-induced breathing patterns like breath-holding, mouth-breathing, yawning, sighing, and rapid, panting-like breathing are, in general, behaviors that we can change. Although breathing is automatic, we can adjust our breathing and, thereby, our minds by slowing and deepening our breathing, reducing our stress levels.

Adding breathing to the Five Tibetan Rites is a two-way flow of benefits. When you breathe optimally, using the full range of upward and downward movement of your diaphragm—the principal muscle for respiration—and the expansion and opening of your intercostal rib muscles, you improve your flexibility, postural alignment, coordination, and balance. Utilizing optimal breathing concepts when practicing the Rites reduces the risk of musculoskeletal strain or injury.

Additionally, the pressure changes from the diaphragm's upward and downward movements help pump lymph throughout the body, boosting the immune system and aiding blood flow back to the heart.

Since breathing optimally is directly linked to your health, well-being, and vitality, Carolinda decided to add breathing to the Rites. However, unlike various breathing exercises and *pranayama* techniques, which often increase tension by design, Carolinda set out to achieve the opposite—loosening and toning the breathing muscles of the body so that a natural, full, sustaining breath could be taken during practice of the Rites and in everyday life.

In this book, Carolinda has achieved what she set out to do. The exercises are simple and easy to follow and apply. Daily practice can improve your lung capacity, slow your breathing rate, and oxygenate your blood. It can reduce stress, boost concentration and mental clarity, improve digestion and absorption of nutrients, and increase your breathing capacity, giving you more energy to do the things you love.

Michael Grant White
Founder, Optimal Breathing Academy
October 2024

AUTHOR'S NOTE

When I began teaching and practicing the Rites over twenty-three years ago, most people were learning the Rites from the simple instructions in the 1939 book, *The Eye of Revelation*, which introduced the Rites to the West.

My workshops attracted a diverse group of people of all ages, backgrounds, abilities, and fitness levels, all seeking to stay fit, youthful, and healthy for longer. Interestingly, many had already attempted to learn the movements from *The Eye of Revelation*. Although charmingly written in the language of its time, the book focuses more on the story behind the Five Tibetan Rites than on providing clear instructions for performing them. As a result, many students needed more detailed guidance to practice the movements confidently, and some required modifications to accommodate injuries, muscle weaknesses, or other limitations.

Many of my students were qualified health practitioners who offered valuable suggestions on reducing strain, preventing injury, and overcoming challenges. After consulting with some of them, I integrated their ideas into my workshops. This collaboration led to the creation of a step-by-step method for mastering the original movements, incorporating core stability strength to protect the spine and natural, full breathing to boost energy and vitality.

Interestingly, despite mindfulness of the breath being an ancient practice integral to Tibetan Buddhist rituals, breathing was not included with the Rites. I was puzzled by its absence, particularly after discovering the author's instructions to "stand with your hands on your hips and take two deep breaths" after each Rite **was removed** from a later version of *The Eye of Revelation* published in 1946.

Intrigued, I conducted a word-by-word, line-by-line comparison of both versions of the book in search of more information. While I didn't find an answer to the missing breathing instructions, I uncovered many fascinating differences, including additional guidance and new insights. These findings are clearly outlined in my comparison book, *The Eye of Revelation 1939 & 1946 Editions Combined*, important extracts of which you can read in full in Part Two.

Understanding how optimal breathing can enhance health and vitality while irregular breathing patterns can have the opposite effect, I decided to reintroduce proper breathing techniques to the Rites. Over the past twenty-three years, students have consistently reported that incorporating breathing into the exercises has increased their enjoyment and improved their daily mood, focus, energy, well-being, and overall sense of joy.

I call the step-by-step method I use to teach the Rites "T5T" (short for The Five Tibetans) to identify it from others, and you will see this term mentioned throughout this book. The integrity of the original Rites remains the same; you get the same benefits but also gain significant additional benefits from core strength development and natural full breathing.

INTRODUCTION

Today, millions of people worldwide are said to practice or have practiced the Five Tibetan Rites. A simple search online will reveal hundreds, if not thousands, of testimonials from people describing how the Five Tibetans have changed their lives—improving physical strength, body tone, flexibility, and health and boosting their energy, well-being, vitality, and happiness.

The benefits are not just physical either; many practitioners claim that practicing the Rites has enabled them to create and do the things they previously lacked the motivation or energy to complete—providing them with a greater sense of achievement, purpose, and fulfillment. Most long-term practitioners say they would never stop practicing them, and I'm one of them.

Learning how to improve your breathing has become very popular in the last decade—it is, after all, essential to life and has many benefits to our health and well-being. In this book, you will learn how combining the benefits of the Rites with the energy-raising benefits of natural full breathing supercharges the benefits of both practices. You will increase awareness of your breathing and improve your health and well-being by learning to breathe slower, easier, and deeper—not only when performing the Rites but in your everyday life, too. Combining breathing with The Five Tibetan Rites seems just "right." It feels great, too.

To help you understand the content better, here is how this book is laid out.

PART 1: BREATHING WITH THE RITES

This section offers straightforward methods to assess and enhance your breathing. You'll engage in exercises designed to explore your breathing patterns and habits. Through this process, you will learn how to incorporate natural, full breathing with The Five Tibetan Rites and in everyday life.

PART TWO: THE BREATHING EXERCISES WITH THE RITES

In this section, you will learn the two breathing techniques that integrate with your Five Tibetan Rites practice: "Energy Breathing," which is carried out three times between each Rite, and "How to Breathe When Practicing The 5 Rites."

PART THREE: THE FIVE TIBETAN RITES

This section covers everything you need to know before practicing the Five Tibetan Rites. You will learn how to perform the exercises using the original instructions from my 1939 and 1946 combined versions of Peter Kelder's book, *The Eye of Revelation,* that introduced the Rites to the West. Drawing on my twenty-three years of teaching experience, I've included extra practice tips, detailed instructions, and guidance on what to avoid and where to focus your attention.

NOTE: None of the information in this book is medical advice. Its purpose is to assist you in breathing easier, slower, and more fully to reduce stress and to provide you with greater energy and well-being by including breathing with The Five Tibetan Rites. If you suffer from any serious breathing difficulties like asthma, COPD, emphysema, or heart disease, please check with your doctor, as is advised, before beginning any new exercise routine, including breathing exercises.

PART ONE

BREATHING
WITH THE RITES

1

STOP
THE CLOCK

T he origins of these five popular anti-aging exercises, known as The Five Tibetan Rites of Rejuvenation, are said to be centuries old—but their ancient source is yet to be discovered. The first mention of the Rites was altogether more modern in a 1939 book called *The Eye of Revelation* by Peter Kelder, which introduced the Rites to the West.

In *The Eye of Revelation,* the central character, a retired British army officer called Colonel Bradford (a pseudonym), was so astounded at the health and vitality of the seemingly ageless monks he discovered that he decided to live and study with them at their remote Tibetan monastery for several years. When he entered the Lamasery, Bradford was "thin and stooped" and leaned heavily on his cane when he walked. Aware of his own aging process, Bradford aimed to stop the clock by discovering the Lama's secrets to the fountain of youth.

Having achieved all he had hoped for, Bradford returned to the US, where he revealed all he had learned to his friend, the author, Peter Kelder. Kelder, who had been expecting Bradford to have aged in the years since they had last met, was "incredulous" at Bradford's transformation into a "tall, straight, ruddy complexioned man in the prime of life."[1]

Bradford explained that he had learned the lamas' secrets to longevity and wellness—to get the body's energy centers spinning again.

"The body has seven centers, which, in English, could be called Vortexes. These are kind of magnetic centers. They revolve at great speed in the healthy body, but when slowed down – well, that is just another name for old age, ill-health, and senility. These spinning centers of activity extend beyond the flesh in the healthy individual, but in the old, weak, senile person, they hardly reach the surface except in the knees. The quickest way to regain health, youth, and vitality is to start these magnetic centers spinning again. There are but five practices that will do this. Any one of them will be helpful, but all five are required to get glowing results. These five exercises are really not exercises at all, in the physical culture sense. The Lamas think of them as 'Rites,' and so instead of calling them exercises or practices, we, too, shall call them 'Rites.'

—**Peter Kelder,** *The Eye of Revelation.*

All efforts to identify and locate either Bradford or Kelder have so far failed (they wouldn't be alive today anyway). However, the legend of the Five Tibetan Rites lives on, gaining strength with the vast numbers of people who learn and practice them globally.

Unfortunately, the likelihood of discovering the remote monastery where the "ageless" monks lived has diminished ever further since the 1950 Chinese invasion of Tibet. Today, only a handful of Tibet's 6,000 Buddhist and Bön monasteries survive.[2] Many thousands of spiritual texts, historical buildings, religious artifacts, and decorative arts are now lost to all of us—perhaps for all time. Of those that survived, many found their way to Dharamsala in India, where the Dalai Lama fled and established his Tibetan Government in Exile.

TRACING HISTORICAL EVIDENCE OF THE FIVE TIBETAN RITES

For many, the story of the Five Tibetan Rites brings to mind ancient spiritual mysteries and hidden secrets of the much-desired fountain of youth. Everyone who has come across the Rites wants to know if they are real and if the benefits claimed for them are true.

According to the publisher of *The Eye of Revelation*, the Rites are 25 centuries old, which places them around the same time as Buddha, who lived in northern India sometime between the 6th and 4th centuries BCE.[3] Buddha, whose real name was Siddhartha Gautama, was born in Lumbini, Nepal, and died when he was around 80 years old. His followers, known as Buddhists, began introducing meditation practices and guidelines for attaining enlightenment in Tibet in the 7th century.

Songsten Gampo, the 33rd Tibetan religious king (crowned 629) of the time, is credited with introducing Buddhism to Tibet. Since Tibet had no writing at the time, Gampo sent one of his ministers to India, who returned with a script (Sanskrit) that was adapted to the Tibetan language.[4] Written records from this period are very scarce since the oral tradition of sharing knowledge from master to student was still in place.[5] Compounding the difficulty for scholars and researchers today is the decomposition of the materials (animal skin, birch bark, palm leaf) they wrote on, such as this Sanskrit palm-leaf scroll from around 828 AD.

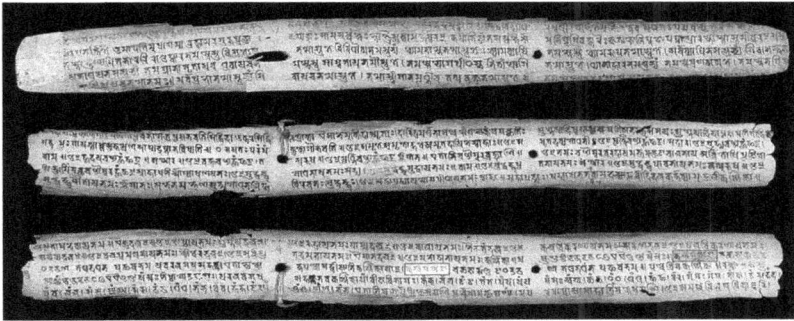

Sanskrit Palm-Leaf Scroll 828 AD – *Wikimedia Commons*[6]

By the end of the 12th Century, Buddhism had largely disappeared from most of India following the Muslim conquests beginning with the Turks. The invaders destroyed Buddhist monasteries, burned their texts, and killed their monks. To escape persecution, Buddhist monks fled to Tibet,[7] where Buddhism still survived. For the next 150 years, commencing around 842 BC, Buddhist and non-Buddhist lineages continued to be studied together.[8]

According to Reginal Ray, author of *Indestructible Truth: The Living Spirituality of Tibetan Buddhism,* "Buddhist teachings, practices, and lineages, particularly tantric ones that did not rely on the court or monastery for their existence, continued to be practiced and passed on from teacher to disciple within individual families and small groups of practitioners." [9]

Some people have speculated that the Rites' origins stem from the minority indigenous Tibetan religion, Bön, which predates Buddhism. Bön retains elements from earlier Tibetan spiritual traditions and is characterized by shamanistic and animist practices, including sacrifices, spells, worship of icons and deities, and mystic rituals. According to noted Tibetologist and historian Per Kværne in his book, *The Bon Religion of Tibet*, "Bön was introduced into Tibet many centuries before Buddhism and enjoyed royal patronage until it was finally supplanted by the 'false religion' (i.e., Buddhism) from India.[10]

It is hard to pinpoint what components of The Five Tibetan Rites are Bön or Hindu-Buddhist practices since Tibetan Buddhism "incorporates the monastic disciplines of early Theravada Buddhism and the shamanistic features of the indigenous Tibetan religion, Bon,"[11] There is no historical evidence of the Rites in either religion so far.

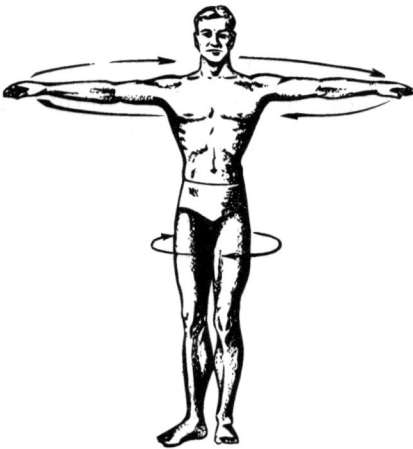

The 1st Rite – The Spin

The first Rite, a spinning movement, is unique, and its origins have intrigued many students over the years. To carry out the spin, you stand upright with your arms spread wide in a T-shape and spin clockwise, building up repetitions until you can do 21 repetitions during your daily practice. The clockwise direction of the spin is perhaps a clue to its Tibetan Buddhist origins. According to the First Dalai Lama (1392-1474), that shortly before his death, the Buddha is said to have remarked, "After my passing away, there will be activities such as circumambulation of these places and reverence to them." [12]

Circumambulation (walking around), known as *Kora* or *Pradakshina*, is still common today. Buddhist pilgrims and followers circumambulate sacred mountains, monasteries, deities, etc., in a clockwise direction—following the sun's movement across the sky.

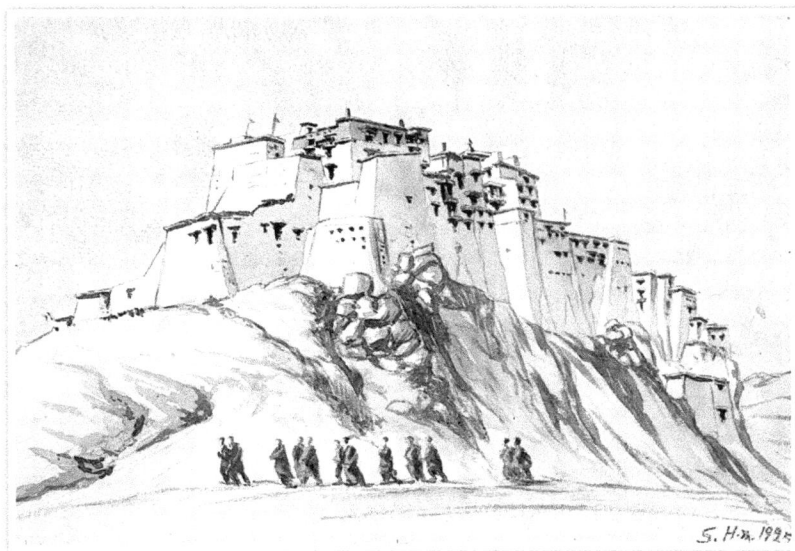

Sven Hedin, Public domain, via Wikimedia [13]

In Bon, pilgrims turn counterclockwise.[14] So do the Turkish Whirling Dervishes, who practice a similar spinning movement (during the *Sema,* a religious ceremony) originating from the 13th Century. They also spin counterclockwise.

Today, as well as historically, many devotional spinning actions are carried out clockwise in Tibet as part of everyday life. Devotees and monks constantly spin handheld prayer wheels with a flick of the wrist or spin huge prayer wheels outside the entrance of temples. Even the mantas inscribed on the outside and written on paper rolls inside the prayer wheels follow a clockwise direction. The purpose of the wheels is to purify negative karma and spread the benefits of the mantras into the environment in all directions.[15] Perhaps the spinning of our body in the first Rite has a similar intention, but that's just speculation on my part.

While no record has been found to confirm the age and origins of the Rites, the opposite is the case for breathing. An ancient Buddhist source that describes Buddha's teaching on the awareness of breathing is a core mindfulness practice still in use today. *The Ānāpānasati Sutta* (*Pāli*) "Breath Mindfulness Discourse," [16] from the *Majjhima Nikāya*—a collection of discourses attributed to the Buddha and his disciples—was composed between the 3rd Century BC and 2nd Century AD.[17]

> *Mindfulness of breathing in and out is of great fruit and of great benefit when cultivated and made much of.*
>
> **—Ānāpānasati Sutta**

If the Rites date from 25 centuries ago, as *The Eye of Revelation* claims, then it seems highly likely that the monks would have practiced some form of breathing mindfulness during their daily rituals. Indeed, since breathing was so integral to Tibetan Buddhist culture in the past, as it is today, linking breathing with the Rites is a natural, if not essential, fit.

PRANA - VIBRANT LIFE FORCE

For millennia, various cultures have recognized the power of breath control as a tool for spiritual enlightenment and a means to enhance health, preserve youthfulness, and extend life. Today, modern science affirms what ancient civilizations intuitively understood: the way you breathe can profoundly impact your longevity. One key measure is "vital capacity," the total volume of air your lungs can hold—a vital indicator of respiratory health and overall well-being.

In Traditional Tibetan Medicine, "the general description of *Lung* [*rlung* pronounced "*loong.*") is that it is a subtle flow of energy, and out of the five elements (air, fire, water, earth, and space), it is most closely connected with air." – Dr. Tamdin Sither Bradley. [18]

In Hindu philosophy, universal life energy, known as *prana*, is believed to be a vital force that permeates everything within and around us. This subtle energy flows through the body via channels called *nadis*. Many cultures have their own names for this essential life force: the Tibetans call it *rlung*, the Chinese know it as *Qi* (or *chi*), the Japanese refer to it as *Ki*, the ancient Greeks called it *Pneuma*, in Polynesian cultures it's known as *Mana*, and in Hebrew, it is called *Ruach*.

Breathing is more than just a physical act of respiration; it is the vibrant life force that enters us at birth and departs at death. The Latin word *spiritus,* meaning "breath of life," reflects this profound connection. As bestselling author Deepak Chopra aptly puts it, "Breathing is the link between the biological and spiritual elements of our nature." Through breath, we bridge the physical and the metaphysical, grounding us in both our human existence and our deeper, spiritual essence."

Prana is the energy permeating the universe at all levels—physical, mental, intellectual, sexual, spiritual, and cosmic energy. It is usually translated as "breath." Thus, pranayama is an art and has techniques to make the respiratory organs move and expand intentionally, rhythmically and intensively.

—**BKS Iyengar**, *Light on Pranayama*

Yogic breathing techniques, known as pranayama, focus on directing the breath to regulate the flow of prana—the vital life force—throughout the body. Prana can be absorbed from everything around us: the sun, sea, air, earth, sacred places, other living beings, the food we eat, and the water we drink. By reconnecting with this original life energy, we can restore our natural ability to heal and rejuvenate both body and spirit.

WHAT HAPPENS WHEN WE BREATHE (MADE SIMPLE)

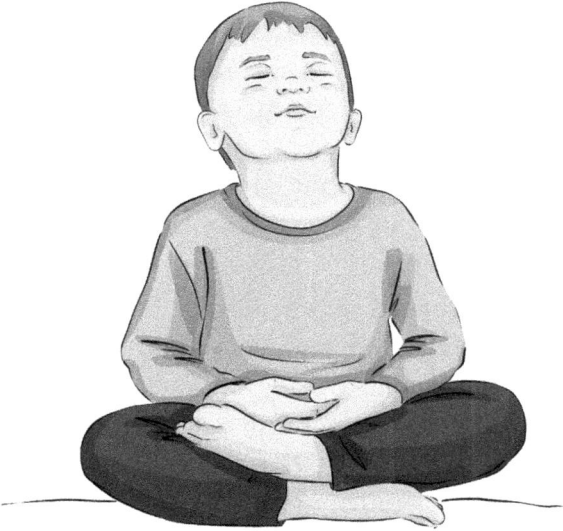

If you've ever built an open fire, you know the more oxygen it receives, the hotter, brighter, and cleaner it burns. With ample oxygen, the fire consumes all the available fuel, mainly leaving ash. However, when oxygen is limited, the fire produces more smoke, generates less heat, and leaves partially burned fuel behind—creating more waste to clean up.

NO OXYGEN = NO ENERGY

When we eat, our bodies digest food and extract nutrients to provide energy. While we can survive days without water and possibly weeks without food, we can't last more than a few minutes without breathing. After digestion, nutrients enter the bloodstream and are transported to the tiny structures in our cells called mitochondria. These mitochondria "burn" oxygen to convert glucose into the energy-carrying molecule called ATP (adenosine triphosphate)—the "fuel of life" that powers every function in our bodies.

Every living organism relies on ATP for energy; without it, we wouldn't have the fuel to sustain life. The more optimal your breathing, the more energy is available for your cells to regenerate and repair. Simultaneously, carbon dioxide—a by-product of this metabolic process—is expelled through respiration, a process just as vital to your health as your bowel and urinary functions.

We breathe constantly, around 12-15 times a minute (17,000 - 22,000 times a day), often without even noticing. Our lungs work tirelessly to bring oxygen into our bloodstream and remove carbon dioxide. From our first breath to our last, they work around the clock, 24 hours a day.

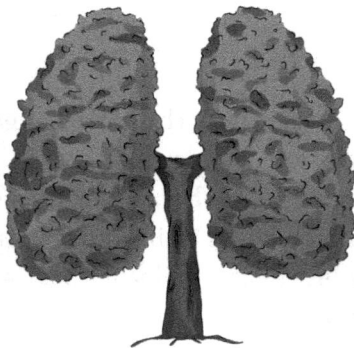

It's fascinating that trees do the opposite of what we do. Through photosynthesis, plants absorb carbon dioxide from the atmosphere, combine it with sunlight and water from the soil, and produce sugars to nourish themselves. The byproduct of this process is oxygen. In a very real sense, we breathe in the oxygen that plants produce, and they "breathe" in the carbon dioxide we exhale. Nature's balance is truly remarkable.

Just as our soul, being air, holds us together, so breath and air encompass the whole world.

—**Anaximenes** (585–528 BCE)

THE PROCESS OF BREATHING MADE SIMPLE

Your lungs, nestled within your ribcage on either side of your heart, are where the vital gas exchange so essential for life occurs. The primary muscles responsible for breathing are the diaphragm—a large dome-shaped muscle beneath your lungs—and the intercostal muscles between each rib.

When you inhale, your diaphragm contracts, lowering and flattening to create more space in your chest cavity, allowing your lungs to expand. The intercostal muscles between your ribs also contract, lifting your rib cage upward and outward, further increasing space for your lungs to expand.

When you breathe out, your diaphragm and rib muscles relax, reducing the space in your chest cavity and causing the lungs to deflate, releasing air like a balloon.

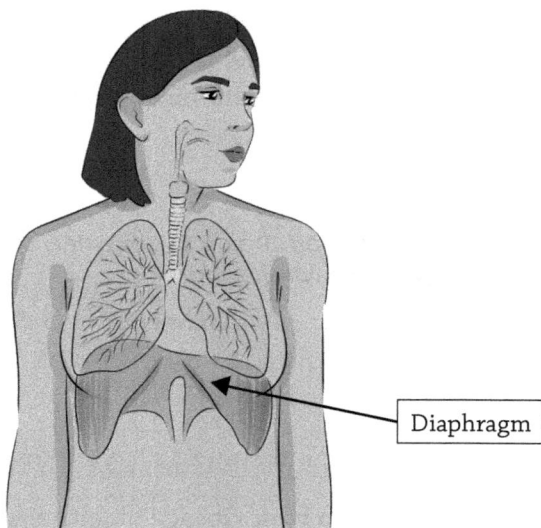

Diaphragm

Your Brain

Your brain regulates breathing in coordination with your respiratory muscles. When it detects low oxygen or high carbon dioxide levels in the blood, it signals the respiratory muscles to adjust the breathing rate (number of breaths per minute) and depth accordingly.

THE VITAL GAS EXCHANGE ESSENTIAL TO LIFE

- **Breathing In** - When you inhale, the concentration of oxygen (O_2) in the lungs is higher than in the blood, causing oxygen to move from the lungs into the bloodstream. Red blood cells in the capillaries surrounding the alveoli (tiny air sacs) in the lungs absorb the oxygen and transport it to the body's cells, where it is used in combination with glucose to produce energy.

- **Breathing Out** - At the same time, carbon dioxide (CO_2), a by-product of metabolism, diffuses from the blood into the alveoli to be exhaled. When you breathe out, the CO_2 concentration is higher in the blood than in the lungs, so CO_2 leaves the bloodstream, enters the alveoli, and is expelled from the body.

THE WAY YOU BREATHE AFFECTS HOW YOU FEEL AND LIVE

3

Although they used different languages and concepts, ancient spiritual traditions recognized that stress and tension disrupted natural breathing patterns, often worsening the problem and deepening suffering. Buddha's followers practiced mindfulness of the breath (*Ānāpānasati*, Pali; Sanskrit) to cultivate spiritual awareness, alleviate suffering, and ultimately attain nirvana (enlightenment). The Buddha's teachings on this practice, passed down through his disciples, date back to approximately the 2nd to 5th century CE. [19] Here is an excerpt below.

Breathing in long, he discerns, "I am breathing in long;" or breathing out long, he discerns, "I am breathing out long." Or breathing in short, he discerns, "I am breathing in short;" or breathing out short, he discerns, "I am breathing out short." He trains himself, "I will breathe in sensitive to the entire body." He trains himself, "I will breathe out sensitive to the entire body." He trains himself, "I will breathe in calming bodily fabrication." He trains himself, "I will breathe out calming bodily fabrication."

—Ānāpānasati Sutta [20]

In Tibetan Medicine, "balance" is defined as the harmony between body, energy, and mind. According to the International Academy for Traditional Tibetan Medicine, "Of these, energy is the most important, as it is the vital link between body and mind. When this vitalizing energy becomes imbalanced, the physical body and the mind also lose their balance, resulting in ill health. Good balance results in a healthy body, a clear, calm mind, and abundant energy." [21]

YIN-YANG AND OUR NERVOUS SYSTEM [22]

For over two thousand years, strong cultural ties and trade have existed between the civilizations of Tibet, India, and China. Each civilization has influenced the others, such as the spread of Buddhist teachings from India to Tibet and the introduction of the yin-yang concept from China during the Tang Dynasty (618–907 CE).

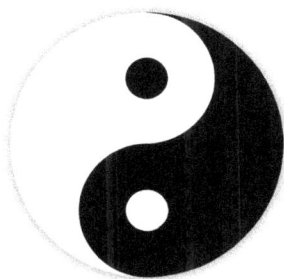

Yin-yang is a fundamental concept in traditional Chinese medicine and philosophy, representing the two complementary forces in creation (e.g., male/female, positive/negative), symbolizing two halves of a unified whole. According to Wan-Chung Hu from the National Research Institute of Chinese Medicine in Taipei, Taiwan, the concept of Yin-Yang in Traditional Chinese Medicine (TCM) can be related to the balance system of our body—specifically the sympathetic and parasympathetic nervous systems. Hu explains, "Yin is related to the parasympathetic system, and Yang is related to the sympathetic system. The antagonism or balance of the two systems can well explain our body's physiological functions." [23]

The sympathetic and parasympathetic nervous systems are key components of the autonomic nervous system, which controls involuntary and reflexive functions, such as breathing and heartbeat. During moments of perceived threat or danger, the sympathetic nervous system takes charge, activating the body's "fight or flight" response. In contrast, the parasympathetic nervous system dominates when you feel safe and calm, promoting "rest and digest" and "feed and breed" functions. Together, these systems maintain balance in the body and ensure survival.

Taking care of your nervous system and body by managing stress, eating a balanced diet, staying physically active, and avoiding drugs and alcohol abuse is essential for overall well-being. I know we've all heard this advice a thousand times, but more recently, there has been growing awareness of the importance of breathing—not just for meditation or mindfulness, but as a key factor in sustaining both physical and mental health.

STRESS AND BREATHING

In today's complex world, most people experience stress and may unknowingly breathe rapidly or shallowly into the upper chest. This type of chest breathing activates the sympathetic nervous system's flight-or-fight response to help you think and act quickly when faced with stress, threats, or danger.

While the fight-or-flight response is crucial in genuine emergencies, remaining in a state of constant sympathetic arousal is detrimental to your health and well-being. As illustrated in the diagram below, prolonged activation of this response can lead to burnout, fatigue, anxiety, nervousness, fear, and sleep disturbances—all symptoms of nervous system exhaustion. Many of us can relate to these effects at some point in our lives.

The parasympathetic nervous system sends signals to relax the body's systems that the sympathetic nervous system has put on alert. Breathing in a regular breathing pattern, slower and deeper into the belly, activates the parasympathetic nervous system's rest-and-digest or feed-and-breed response—directly impacting your emotions, helping you handle stress better, increasing your energy, and improving your health. Slower breathing also lengthens your lifespan.[24]

THE MAIN DIFFERENCES BETWEEN THE SYMPATHETIC AND PARASYMPATHETIC NERVOUS SYSTEMS		
	Sympathetic (flight-or-fight response).	Parasympathetic (rest-and-digest or feed-and-breed response).
Pupils	*Your pupils widen to allow more light into your eyes so you can see better and further.*	*The size of your pupils decreases, and your close-up vision improves.*
Breathing	*Your breathing rate increases, and your airways widen to allow more oxygen intake.*	*Your breathing rate slows, and your airways narrow slightly as your body requires less oxygen.*
Heart	*Increases heart rate and blood pressure to direct blood flow to vital organs and muscles.*	*Your heart rate slows to a resting rate, and your blood pressure lowers.*
Digestion	*Your digestive system slows down so the energy can be diverted to other body parts.*	*Stimulates digestion. Increases saliva production and gastric secretions and activates peristalsis in the gut.*

Kidney, Liver & bladder	*Your kidneys release adrenaline to prepare you for action, and your liver releases glucose for energy. Your bladder relaxes, inhibiting urination.*	*Helps counteract the effects of adrenaline and bring the body back to a state of balance (homeostasis). Informs the pancreas to produce insulin to break down sugars. Contracts your bladder so you can pee.*
Sexual Function	*Triggers ejaculation and orgasm. Overactivation, especially from stress or anxiety, can inhibit sexual performance.*	*Initiates sexual arousal and lubrication by increasing localized blood flow.*
Mood	*Produces feelings of stress, anxiety, fear, or nervousness to help you fight or escape from a threat or stress.*	*Produces a calming and relaxing effect on your mood.*
Immune System	*Shift resources away to focus on immediate survival.*	*Improves immune system activity for healing and recovery.*

Your breath is the first function of the body to be affected by how you feel, so don't expect your breathing to have the same pattern every day. Whatever happens in the mind influences the breath. Through daily awareness of your breathing, you can gradually reverse this process, as changing your breathing pattern can influence your mind. In other words—to *BE* calm, *BREATHE* calmly.

Breathing in, I calm body and mind. Breathing out, I smile. Dwelling in the present moment, I know this is the only moment.

—Thich Nhat Hanh, *Vietnamese Buddhist monk*

HOW WELL YOU BREATHE CAN PREDICT YOUR LIFESPAN

Clinical studies have proven that how well you breathe affects your lifespan.[25] Researchers from The Framingham Heart Study, a long-term, ongoing cardiovascular study that began in 1948, now on its third generation of participants, could foretell how long a person would live by measuring forced exhalation breathing (FEVI) volume and hypertension (high blood pressure).[26] Forced expiratory volume calculates the amount of air that a person can force out of their lungs in one second.

William B. Kannel of the Boston School of Medicine (1981), a former director of the Framingham study, states, "We know that much of hypertension is controlled by the way we breathe. Long before a person becomes terminally ill, vital capacity can predict life span." Vital capacity (a typical adult's vital capacity is between 3 – 5 liters) is the maximum amount of air a person can expel from the lungs after being filled completely.[27]

According to the American Lung Foundation, your lungs mature by the time you are about 20-25 years old. After around 35, it is normal for your lung function to decline gradually as you age—due to decreased elasticity, weakened respiratory muscles, and a stiffer chest wall. By age 65, you've typically lost up to a liter of lung capacity compared with when you were younger.[28] This can make breathing slightly more difficult as you age, but if you notice any sudden breathing difficulties or shortness of breath, talk to your doctor straight away, as this may be related to a health condition.

To improve lung and heart efficiency, the American Lung Association recommends 30 minutes of moderate physical activity five days a week, with the following guidelines to help achieve this.

- Strengthen and tone your diaphragm and intercostal muscles through exercises like diaphragmatic (belly) breathing, such as the Energy Breathing Technique, which you'll practice between each of the 5 Rites. Singing is another effective way to develop lung capacity and strengthen your breathing muscles. [29]

- Improve your posture so your breathing isn't restricted by poor postural habits like slouching or hunching over. Lung capacity is optimal when you are standing or sitting in a balanced upright position, and your core muscles are strong. That's why strength-building exercises such as the Five Tibetan Rites (particularly the core strength emphasis in the T5T version), weightlifting, and Pilates help build core strength, increase flexibility, and improve posture.

- Engage in activities like brisk walking, swimming, running, cycling, or even vigorous house cleaning to enhance lung function and boost heart and lung efficiency.

- Keep active, as this boosts mental well-being by reducing anxiety and depression and enhancing memory.[30]

For further resources, training, and products to improve lung function, see Further Information at the back of the book.

EXPLORING HOW YOU BREATHE
Breathing rate – How Fast You Breathe

> **NOTE:** *This exercise is not a medical test. If you have existing health issues, physical, mental, or both, and you would like to know what your breathing rate is, you should discuss this with your doctor or qualified health professional.*

Current medical opinion is that 12 to 20 breaths per minute is considered normal.[31] Michael Grant White, founder of Optimal Breathing, whose normal breathing rate is 8 and resting rate is 6, believes that "normal" is neither optimal nor healthy. White claims that unless your breathing rate is already low, you can definitely benefit from slowing down your breathing—and that regular practice of T5T's breathing exercises can help you achieve this.

In a fascinating study that tested whether external rhythms could influence internal ones, Dr. Luciano Bernadi and Associates from the University of Pavia, Italy, stated in *Circulation,* the journal of the American Heart Association, that "If, instead of breathing naturally, you superimpose a slow, steady rate of respiration on the body, you modulate (regulate) the whole cardiovascular system." [32]

The results of this study using rhythmic formulas such as reciting the *Ave Maria* (in Latin) and yoga mantras caused striking, powerful, and synchronous increases in existing cardiovascular rhythms when recited at 6 breaths per minute.[33] A further study by Dr Bernadi and his Associates concluded "that practicing slow and deep breathing thus can be beneficial in heart failure or in other diseases." [34]

Try the following exercise to determine your breathing rate when you are fully relaxed. It's simple: count the number of breaths you take by observing how many times your chest or abdomen rises over the course of one minute. However, make sure you are entirely relaxed before starting, as even a short walk across the room can elevate your breathing rate.

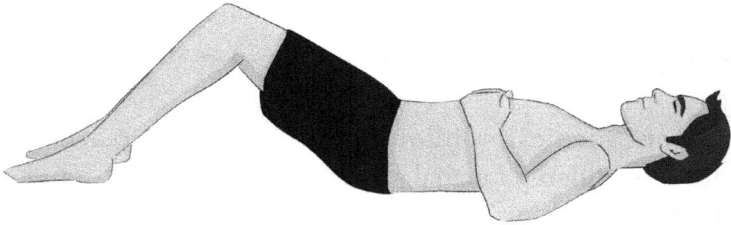

EXERCISE

Set your mobile phone, watch, or other timer for one minute. When you are ready, press start. Stop when one minute is over. If you don't have a suitable device to time yourself, ask someone to help you.

- Sit or lie down and try to relax.
- When you feel relaxed, press start on your timer.
- Count the number of times your chest or abdomen rises over the course of one minute.
- Remember this number when the minute is up—this is your breathing rate per minute.
- If you are unsure of the count, repeat the test two or three times or until the number of breaths is identical (or nearly).

Our breathing naturally adjusts to our circumstances, so a higher breathing rate doesn't necessarily indicate a problem. Various factors, such as your current health, anxiety, mood changes, injuries, illness, digestion, alcohol consumption, physical exercise, or underlying conditions, can affect your breathing rate. Even the stress of worrying about how to carry out the test or what result you obtain can influence it.

If you were in a medical setting, an atypical respiratory rate, especially if it is too fast, could indicate a health problem.[35]

When you have been practicing T5T for a few months, repeat the test and see if there is any difference.

THE RELATIONSHIP BETWEEN EMOTIONS & BREATHING

Have you noticed that your breathing naturally slows down when you're relaxed, and when you're nervous or anxious, it speeds up? Have you ever tried intentionally slowing your breath during stressful moments and felt calmer as a result? Numerous studies have shown that altering our breathing patterns can significantly influence our emotional state, reinforcing the strong connection between breathing and mood.[36]

Researchers at the Institute for Physiology at the University of Freiburg, Germany,[37] concluded that there is a strong reciprocal relationship between emotions and respiration. Their study, conducted in two parts, examined the impact of rhythmic breathing on brain activity across a range of emotions.

- In the first part, participants were asked to experience various emotions and describe their breathing patterns during those emotional states.

- In the second part, participants were given a cover story to mask the study's purpose and instructed to follow specific breathing patterns designed to evoke significant emotional responses.

- The researchers found that certain breathing patterns were consistently linked to similar emotional states across all participants.

So, the next time you feel anxious or stressed, check if your breathing has become rapid and shallow; then, make sure you are breathing through your nose and begin to slow your breathing rate—like this:

Slow Down Your Breathing Rate

- Place one hand on your upper chest and one on your belly just below your ribcage.
- Breathe only through your nose.
- Then, begin to breathe slower and deeper into your abdomen. The hand on your belly will begin to rise higher than the one on your chest.
- Relax any tension in your shoulders and focus on increasing the length of your exhalation.
- Allow yourself to experience a pause after exhalation, allowing the inhalation to arrive by itself naturally.
- Repeat until you feel your breathing slows and your mind becomes calm.

Continue in this manner until you feel more relaxed—then smile. Smiling releases endorphins and helps manage stress. Try it, it works!

Later in this chapter, you can also try the Exercises to Calm Your Mind.

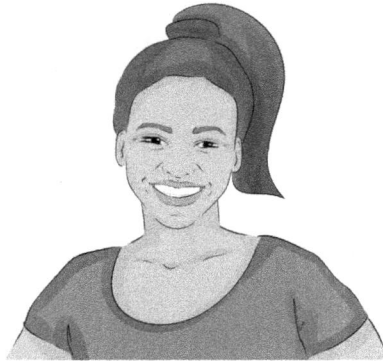

> "Sometimes your joy is the source of your smile, but sometimes your smile can be the source of your joy."
>
> —**Thich Nhat Hanh**, *Vietnamese Buddhist monk*

SELF-REFLECTION AND CHANGE

The way we breathe reflects how we respond to situations, what brings us joy, and what we avoid. As our breath passes through our vocal cords, it allows us to express our thoughts, passions, joys, and knowledge. How we breathe is, in essence, how we live—whether we rush through life taking short, rapid breaths, sipping in tiny bits of air, or breathing in fully and embracing life itself.

Becoming mindful of your breathing and developing an awareness of how your breath moves through your body can be a transformative tool for self-reflection and change. For instance, the next time you catch yourself breathing rapidly into your chest, pause and ask yourself what you're experiencing at that moment. Are you feeling stressed, anxious, or rushed? Try slowing down your breathing and observe whether the tension starts to ease. This simple act of mindfulness—pausing, questioning, and intentionally slowing your breath—can make stress more manageable and lead to profound changes in your emotional well-being and overall quality of life.

The following exercises are simple to practice and are highly effective in calming and centering your mind.

> *"Feelings come and go like clouds in a windy sky. Conscious breathing is my anchor."*
>
> — **Thich Nhat Hanh,** *Vietnamese Buddhist monk*

EXERCISES TO CALM YOUR MIND

Pregnant women and individuals who have high blood pressure, heart issues, or respiratory problems should talk to their doctor before carrying out the exercises. Avoid performing the exercises too forcefully or holding your breath for extended periods.

The Humming Breath

This exercise activates the rest-and-digest response of your body. Choose a quiet, calm place where you feel comfortable and relaxed.

- Sit on an upright chair, looking straight ahead, with your shoulders back and your spine straight.
- Close your eyes. Bring your awareness to your breathing and take two normal breaths.

- Place your index fingers or thumbs on the small cartilage protrusions (tragi) near the gateway to your ear canals. Don't stick your fingers in your ears—just press the top of each tragus gently inwards to block off any external sound.
- Take a full breath in through your nose for three seconds.
- Breathe out slowly through your nose and start humming like a bee while gently pressing the tragi to close your ears. You will feel the humming sensation at the back of your nose and throat.
- Repeat the last two steps for 5 breaths to 10 breaths.

Box breathing is a highly recommended technique known for its calming effects, making it ideal for moments of stress or overwhelm. While it isn't a natural breathing pattern, it serves as a temporary method to soothe your mind and reduce tension before returning to your regular breathing rhythm.

If you experience lightheadedness or dizziness during the exercise, shorten the breath-holding intervals and gradually increase them as you feel more comfortable.

The Box Breath (or Square Breath)

You can perform this breathing exercise sitting, standing, or lying. To begin, sit upright on a comfortable chair with your feet on the floor, your shoulders relaxed, and your spine straight.

1. Close your eyes and take a few normal breaths, ending on an exhalation.

2. Breathe in through your nose for a count of 4, expanding your belly and ribs as you do so.

3. Hold the air in your lungs for a count of 4. Try to avoid clamping your mouth or nose shut. (If counting to 4 feels challenging, start with a count of 3 and gradually build up to 4.)

4. Exhale slowly through your nose for a count of 4, allowing your belly and ribs to return to their normal position (without pulling your belly inwards).

5. Hold your lungs empty for a count of 4.

6. Inhale and repeat these steps for around four minutes or until you feel a sense of calm and improved mental focus.

5

GOOD VS. POOR BREATHING

I n recent years, breathing improvement techniques have gained widespread popularity as a path to better health and well-being. With numerous methods, techniques, instructors, and experts available, the options seem vast and sometimes overwhelming. Determining which approach is best suited for us individually can be complex.

The breathing techniques you're about to learn are simple yet powerful, having been tested by thousands of people over the last twenty-three years. They integrate seamlessly into your daily Five Tibetan Rites practice, providing a solid foundation for a deeper exploration of breathwork should you wish to go further.

Michael Grant White, founder of Optimal Breathing, became my go-to expert after I had completed several of his courses and worked with him in private sessions. With over forty years of experience teaching and researching breathing techniques, Mike's expertise is extensive and well-established. Like many other breathing instructors, he emphasizes that we can all improve our breathing by establishing a regular, rhythmic pattern, slowing our breathing rate, taking fuller and deeper breaths, and expanding the flexibility and capacity of our respiratory system.

These outcomes are the cornerstones of T5T's breathing techniques. Students who consistently practice these methods report being able to handle life's challenges with greater clarity, calm, and control. Many also describe improved mental and physical well-being, increased energy levels, and a heightened awareness of non-optimal breathing patterns—with the ability to change them as required.

Breathing slower, deeper, and easier is vital for longevity, health, and vitality. T5T can help most people become more conscious of their breathing. It can also release tension in their breathing, and often gradually expand their breathing capacity as well as slow their breathing rate.

—**Michael Grant White,** Optimal Breathing

ADAPTIVE NATURAL BREATHING

Our breathing is adaptive—there's no single method that suits every situation. Ideally, your breathing should naturally and effortlessly adjust to your activity and environment. Sometimes, your body needs more oxygen, such as during intense exercise or in moments of danger. Stress, or even thinking about stressful situations, can also alter your breathing. At other times, such as when you're relaxing or listening to calming music, your body requires much less oxygen. When you stop to think about it, the fact that your breathing rate, depth, and rhythm adjust naturally according to your activity—that's called living!

You don't need to be relaxed to breathe well—in fact, staying relaxed in situations like facing danger could be harmful. Likewise, belly breathing isn't always necessary and can sometimes lead to overbreathing. Ideally, your breathing should have the capacity, flexibility, and strength to adjust optimally based on the situation at hand.

This is where your brain plays a key role. It regulates your breathing, adjusting both the rate and depth based on signals received from sensors throughout your body, ensuring that your breathing aligns with your needs.

- **Sensors in your lungs** detect irritants, causing your airways to become smaller in response or by making you sneeze or cough to expel them from your body.
- **Sensors in your joints and muscles** detect movement in your arms and legs, sending signals to your brain to adjust your breathing rate and depth in response to your physical activity.
- **Sensors in your brain** detect your blood's carbon dioxide and oxygen levels and trigger respiration in response.[38]

WHAT IS GOOD BREATHING?

When instructed to take a deep breath, many people stand rigid, suck their stomachs in, thrust their chests forward, and forcefully inhale through pinched nostrils while lifting their shoulders. This approach not only sounds exhausting but also restricts breathing by increasing tension throughout the body. Pulling the stomach inwards forces the breath into the chest, limiting the amount of oxygen you can obtain—and is the opposite of what a true deep breath should be—relaxed, expansive, and satisfying.

When you breathe correctly, your entire body "breathes." Like a wave, your breath flows through you, expanding with each inhalation and releasing with each exhalation. Optimal breathing occurs when you effortlessly inhale and exhale fully, providing your body with the right amount of oxygen while efficiently removing waste gases. It engages the full range of motion in your diaphragm, belly, ribs, sides, back, and chest, which adjusts naturally to your oxygen needs.

> *"My experience has taught me that the optimal characteristics are volume, efficiency, strength, balance, and flexibility. Volume is my first priority, then balance. The rest may be related to the task at hand."*
>
> — **Michael Grant White,** Optimal Breathing.

OPTIMAL BREATHING

When breathing optimally explains breathing expert Anders Olsson, founder of The Conscious Breathing Institute, "Inhalation lasts for 2-3 seconds, exhalation for 3-4 seconds, followed by a pause that lasts 2-3 seconds." A good rule of thumb, he says, is "3-3-3." [39]

Michael Grant White says the optimal breathing window is to inhale to 80% of your capacity and breathe out 30% with a pause of about 1-2 seconds before your next inhalation. However, your breathing patterns, health, location, altitude, state of mind, and level of activity will all affect your breathing, so these figures are just a guide.

Don't expect your breathing to have the same pattern every day, as your breath is the first function of the body to be affected by how you feel. Whatever happens in the body and the mind influences the breath. Through daily awareness of your breathing, you can begin to change non-optimal breathing patterns and, in the process, change how you react and grow. For example: To BE calm, BREATHE calm.

Breathe is the bridge which connects life to consciousness, which unites your body to your thoughts. Whenever your mind becomes scattered, use your breath as the means to take hold of your mind again.

—**Thich Nhat Hanh,** Vietnamese Buddhist monk

NON-OPTIMAL BREATHING

Over time, most of us develop poor breathing habits, such as holding our breath when stressed or breathing too much, too little, too fast, or too slow. These habits, which can develop from stress, anxiety, or health issues, are dysfunctional breathing patterns that reduce the efficiency of respiration, creating stress and tension in both body and mind. This can lead to physical and emotional health issues such as fatigue, dizziness, and heightened anxiety.

The good news is that unless you have underlying mental and physical health conditions, you can restore healthy breathing by learning effective techniques such as diaphragmatic breathing, nose breathing, and mindfulness. These techniques are integral to your breathing practice with the Five Tibetan Rites, helping you shift from unconscious autopilot to conscious control.

While breathing exercises can improve many irregular patterns, it is important to recognize when professional care is needed. The following information on non-optimal breathing patterns is not medical advice. If irregular breathing patterns persist despite efforts to correct them or if symptoms worsen (e.g., chest pain, wheezing, fainting), it is essential to consult a healthcare provider. A doctor can conduct specialized tests to determine the underlying cause and recommend appropriate treatment.

Below are some common poor breathing habits, with some suggestions at the end of the chapter on how to change them.

Improper breathing is a common cause of ill health.

— **Dr. Andrew Weil**

Breath Holding

Many people hold their breath when concentrating intensely, like working on the computer or during stressful moments. Breath-holding is also part of the body's fight-or-flight response, where muscles tense, and breathing becomes irregular as the body prepares to respond to perceived threats. We often hold our breath when we anticipate or experience pain during a medical procedure or injury as a protective attempt to alleviate discomfort. Breath-holding can also act as a coping mechanism, often used consciously or unconsciously, to suppress intense emotions such as anger, fear, or sadness.

Frequent, often unconscious breath-holding can result from stress or anxiety and lead to irregular oxygen exchange. This may cause dizziness, fatigue, poor sleep, and increased anxiety, creating a vicious cycle that keeps the body in a heightened state of alertness.

Reverse breathing

Some people develop a habit known as reverse breathing, where they mistakenly pull their stomachs in while inhaling. Pulling your stomach in (or pushing it out) is unnecessary, as it doesn't aid breathing—it restricts it. The proper way to breathe is as follows: When you inhale, your diaphragm lowers and flattens, pressing down on the abdominal contents and causing them to expand outward. Pulling your stomach in at this point prevents the diaphragm from fully descending, limiting oxygen intake and confining the breath to your chest.

When you exhale, there's no need to pull your stomach inward, as exhalation is a passive process whereby your breathing muscles naturally relax, expelling air from your lungs. Pulling the stomach inward is only necessary during forced exhalation to help push air out more strongly.

Shallow (Chest) breathing

If you frequently yawn, sigh, or take sudden gasps for air, you may be experiencing air hunger. This sensation is a form of incomplete respiration, often stemming from chest or shallow breathing, that occurs when the diaphragm doesn't fully engage, preventing it from descending properly. Instead, air is pulled into the upper chest through quick, shallow breaths, reducing the effectiveness of both inhalation and exhalation. This pattern limits oxygen intake and can cause carbon dioxide retention, making it difficult to feel satisfied with each breath.

Shallow breathing is frequently associated with stress, anxiety, and poor breathing habits. Under stress, individuals may unconsciously shift to this pattern, activating the sympathetic nervous system and triggering a fight-or-flight response. When this occurs, the body remains in a state of heightened alertness, which can worsen anxiety and perpetuate the cycle of shallow breathing and emotional stress. Learning diaphragmatic breathing (as you are about to do) can help restore proper breathing, reduce stress, promote relaxation, and help break the anxiety and shallow breathing cycle.

Overbreathing (hyperventilation)

Breathing more rapidly or deeply than the body's metabolic needs can lead to excess oxygen intake and a drop in carbon dioxide levels, impairing the body's ability to use oxygen effectively. When carbon dioxide levels decrease, your blood vessels constrict, reducing blood flow and limiting oxygen delivery throughout your body. This imbalance between oxygen and carbon dioxide—known as hyperventilation—can result in symptoms such as lightheadedness, tingling sensations, and an increased heart rate. It's important to distinguish between healthy deep breathing (which can be calming and beneficial) and hyperventilation, which can trigger anxiety and other physical symptoms.

Hyperventilation can also result from a sudden panic response, such as during panic attacks, or be triggered by injury, trauma, extreme stress, phobias, or fear. Respiratory conditions like asthma or COPD, certain medications (such as sedatives or anesthetics), high altitudes, or hot weather can also contribute to hyperventilation.

Monitoring Your Breathing Patterns

Regular practice of The Five Tibetan Rites, combined with mindful breathing, enhances your awareness of non-optimal breathing patterns. Once identified, you can intentionally shift to a more rhythmic, balanced, and fuller breath. The table below is designed to help you track what you were doing when your breathing wasn't optimal, making it easier to identify and understand your patterns. Tracking your progress in the early stages reinforces this awareness and helps you notice subtle changes over time.

Mouth Breathing	When walking.	During sleep. Snoring.
Sighing	After a meeting with my boss.	Sitting at my desk. At least 6 x today.
Yawning	Multiple times at work and during my commute.	When I intensely focus and don't leave my desk.
Holding Breath	All the time when writing emails.	During most of my phone calls.
An urge to take a deep breath	Random 4 x today.	5 x today.
Underbreathing - Shallow Breathing	Social event.	On a date.
Chest Breathing – rapid, shallow breathing	During a team meeting.	Argument with my partner.
Pulling the stomach in or pushing it out	Random 8 x today.	At the Gym.
Balanced, easy Breathing	Watching TV. Hugging my dog.	Reading my book before sleep.

If you create a similar table, keep it nearby to log any changes in your breathing patterns throughout the day. Note the activity or situation you were engaged in at the time, as this will help you identify patterns and triggers—such as specific situations, people, or activities—that influence your breathing. Tracking these habits over a week will help build awareness, allowing you to adjust your breathing or modify activities that contribute to ineffective breathing patterns.

If you have observed a rapid breathing rate and want to slow it down—try the **Slow Down Your Breathing Rate** or one of the **Exercises to Calm Your Mind** in Chapter 4. These exercises are also helpful if you are holding your breath. The **Energy Breathing** technique you are about to learn can also help slow down your breathing. It is also well-suited to deepen and replenish your breathing if you are shallow breathing and can help correct a reverse breathing pattern.

6

PREPARATION FOR THE T5T BREATHING EXERCISES

Suppose you think of the eternal knot, an ancient Tibetan symbol illustrated below, as a guidepost for your journey. It represents the interweaving of wisdom and method, showing how insight and effort work together to create meaningful progress. Similarly, the practices you'll explore here are designed to help you cultivate understanding and practical application, allowing these elements to support each other throughout your experience.

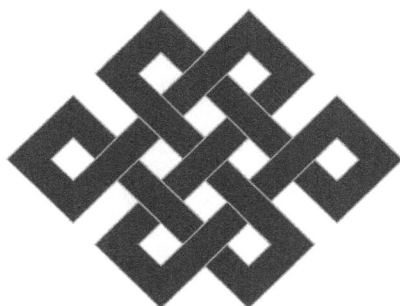

40

The key to improving your breathing during your Five Tibetan Rites practice lies in the understanding you will gain from the preparation exercises below. Just as you can't truly know what chocolate tastes like until you try it—you can't fully understand where the breath moves in your body (or where it doesn't) until you experience it firsthand. Without this understanding, your knowledge may remain superficial.

It's natural to want to rush toward the main goal, but remember that what you're about to learn is a skill that will enhance your vital capacity and overall zest for life. Don't be discouraged by a few anatomical terms—you don't need to be an expert— you just need a basic understanding to benefit fully from these exercises.

ESSENTIAL CONCEPTS BEFORE LEARNING THE 5 RITES

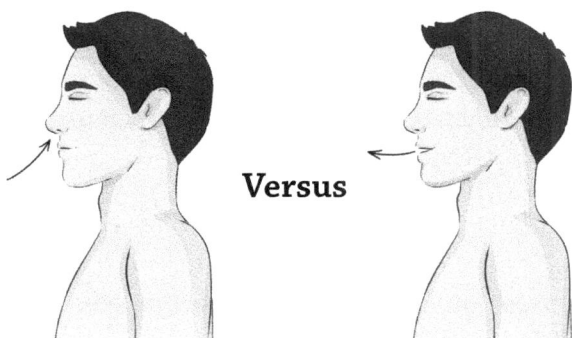

Versus

MOUTH BREATHING VERSUS NOSE BREATHING

While practicing The Five Tibetan Rites, you will breathe only through your nose. Nose breathing slows your breathing naturally by creating resistance. This helps your diaphragm engage and draws oxygen deeper into the lungs. It also slows exhalation, giving your body more time to absorb oxygen into the bloodstream.

Nasal breathing helps maintain the lungs' elasticity, ensuring the best uptake of oxygen and release of Carbon Dioxide,[41] whereas mouth breathing promotes shallow chest breathing, limiting oxygen uptake. Nose breathing plays a vital role in helping regulate carbon dioxide levels in the body, which is essential for maintaining blood pH, widening blood vessels, and ensuring efficient oxygen delivery.

Interestingly, it's not a lack of oxygen but the increased concentration of carbon dioxide in the blood that primarily triggers the urge to breathe.[42] When CO2 levels rise, the brain signals the body to breathe more deeply or rapidly to restore balance. Conversely, when the carbon dioxide levels are low, the brain decreases the frequency and depth of breathing.

Breathing through your nose forces you to slow down, reducing stress and tension. It cleans and filters the air by trapping viruses, bacteria, allergens, and other particles in the cilia (tiny, hairlike structures), provides a sense of smell, and warms and moistens the air so it can move comfortably into your lungs—an average mouth breather bypasses this.

Your nose is designed for breathing, and your mouth is designed for eating.

—Anonymous

Mouth Breathing

Mouth breathing is less efficient than nose breathing and occurs naturally during activities such as singing, shouting, intense exercise, or when you're congested from a cold. It also happens when the body demands more air, such as during extreme fear, stress, or panic. Mouth breathing draws in large volumes of air quickly, but it primarily fills the upper chest, triggering the body's fight-or-flight response and increasing stress and anxiety.

Many people breathe through their mouths without even realizing it, particularly during sleep, which can reduce oxygen levels, disrupt restful sleep, and contribute to snoring. The first step to changing this non-optimal breathing pattern is to become aware of when it happens. Once you notice it, you can gradually adjust your breathing habits by practicing nasal breathing during the day, which may also improve nighttime breathing over time. Please see Further Information at the back of the book for methods to enhance nose breathing during sleep.

Nitric Oxide (NO)

The respiratory cycle is based on the coordinated transport of three gases: nitric oxide, oxygen, and carbon dioxide.[43]

—Professor J. S. Stamler

One of the key benefits of nose breathing is the production of nitric oxide (NO), a molecule that dilates blood vessels and enhances oxygen delivery throughout the body. Despite the significance of nitric oxide's role in respiratory health being backed by research, it is not widely known outside medical or scientific communities.

When you breathe through your nose (but not your mouth), the air mixes with nitric oxide—a natural gas produced in the paranasal sinuses and throughout the body. Nitric oxide plays a crucial role in the immune system by defending against infections, bacteria, and viruses. Additionally, research shows that nitric oxide regulates the release of oxygen from red blood cells into tissues, ensuring that oxygen reaches the areas that need it most.[44]

Since mouth breathing bypasses nitric oxide production in the nasal passages, it reduces the efficiency of oxygen uptake and the body's ability to fight off infections. This makes nasal breathing more beneficial for overall respiratory health.

NOSE BREATHING	MOUTH BREATHING
Warms, cleans and humidifies the incoming air.	Unfiltered, cold, or dry air.
Filters out germs, bacteria, and particles.	Lack of protection due to unfiltered air.
Enables you to smell enticing aromas and warns against harmful odors.	Limited sense of smell—similar to when you have a cold and food tastes bland.
Nitric oxide released in the nasal airways widens blood vessels and improves oxygen absorption.	Depletes carbon dioxide levels. Reduces oxygen absorption.
Encourages satisfying deep (as opposed to big) breaths.	Reduces the diaphragm's range of motion, limiting breathing capacity.
It calms the body and mind and stimulates the body's rest-and-digest response.	Promotes shallow chest breathing, which activates the flight-or-fight response, increasing stress and anxiety.
Increases oxygen uptake.	Less oxygen is available.
Promotes better sleep with less wakefulness and reduced snoring.	Disrupts sleep, causing snoring, wakefulness, and dry mouth.

One Nostril Blocked More Than The Other

Have you ever noticed that one nostril sometimes feels more congested, only for the sensation to switch to the other nostril later? This phenomenon is known as the nasal cycle, a natural process regulated by the autonomic nervous system. In most healthy adults, one nostril becomes more congested while the other clears every four to six hours. Dr. Michael Benninger from the Cleveland Clinic explains that about 75% of our breathing happens through one nostril at a time. Although the exact purpose is unclear, a common theory is that this cycle helps keep the nasal passages moist and prevents them from drying out. [45]

To Clear Your Nose, Try This Exercise

Try this exercise, which encourages your nasal passages to open naturally. After you have completed it, continue to breathe slowly through your nose to maintain the benefits. You can also try the Humming Breath exercise in Chapter 4, which helps with sinus and stress relief.

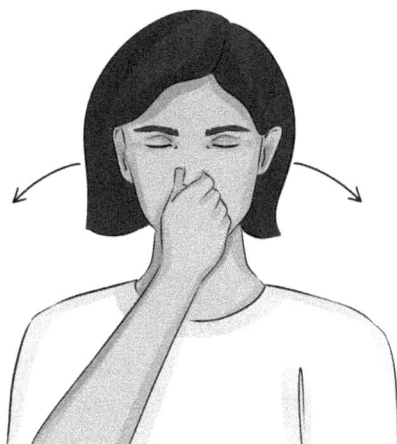

NOTE: *Since this exercise involves holding your breath for a short while, pregnant women and those who suffer from high blood pressure, serious health, or breathing conditions should check with their qualified health practitioner before carrying out this exercise.*

WIDEN YOUR NASAL PASSAGES

You can perform this breathing exercise sitting, standing, or lying.

1. Sit on a straight-backed chair with your spine upright and your feet flat on the floor. Ensure your shoulders are back and relaxed and your head is upright, looking straight ahead.

2. Take two normal breaths in and out through your nose.

3. Exhale fully through your nose, then gently pinch your nose closed at the end of the out-breath.

4. With your mouth closed, slowly nod your head up and down (or sway side to side) while continuing to hold your breath.

5. When you feel a moderate to strong urge to breathe, calmly inhale through your nose.

6. Continue breathing calmly and steadily through your nose for a few minutes. Notice if your nasal breathing feels easier. If not, breathe normally for a minute, then repeat the exercise 2 to 5 more times.

Changing A Mouth Breathing Habit

As you become more mindful of your breathing, you may notice how often you breathe through your nose during the day and night. If you snore, it's often a sign of mouth breathing. To shift this habit, consciously practice nose breathing during the day.

Be patient—a few minutes of daily practice can create lasting improvements over time.

If your nose often feels blocked (or you are getting constant complaints about snoring), consider using a nasal dilator to gently widen your nostrils, making it easier to breathe and sleep. These small, comfortable devices fit inside the nose, holding the airways open, even during deep inhales and exhales.

> **Try this:** *Close your mouth and place the index fingers of both hands on either side of your nose, then gently spread the fingers outward. Is that easier to breathe?*

You could also try using mouth tapes such as MyoTape or similar products at night that encourage nasal breathing and eliminate loud snoring. You will find a list of suppliers and resources at the back of the book.

USING YOUR DIAPHRAGM

During your Five Tibetans practice, you will use your diaphragm to breathe fully, energizing your movements in a flowing, synchronized breathing pattern. Since your lungs are spongy and cannot draw in air on their own, they rely on the diaphragm, a dome-shaped muscle, and other respiratory muscles to do the work. As the diaphragm moves up and down in your chest, it causes the lungs to expand on the in-breath and contract on the out-breath, enabling effective oxygen exchange. It is the primary muscle of your respiration.

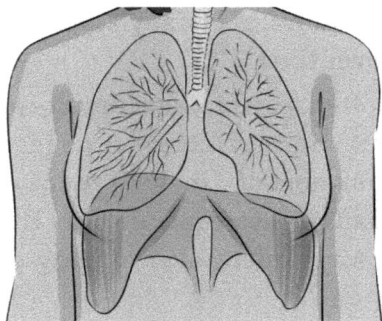

Your diaphragm needs to stay flexible and responsive to ensure your body receives enough oxygen. When the diaphragm isn't functioning optimally, you may rely more on rapid, shallow chest breathing, which triggers the body's fight-or-flight response, increasing tension, stress, and low-level anxiety. Over time, chronic shallow breathing into the upper chest can limit the range of motion in your diaphragm, reducing its efficiency.

The phrase, "If you don't use it, you lose it (until you work on it again)," applies to all muscles, including the diaphragm. Just like other muscles, the diaphragm needs consistent activation to maintain strength and functionality. Restoring full diaphragmatic movement requires conscious practice to re-train your body to breathe deeply and efficiently, helping to reduce stress and restore balance in your nervous system.

Understanding how your diaphragm works allows you to to visualize what happens when you breathe deeply and fully—and when you don't. Since the diaphragm has a dome-like shape, visualizing it as an umbrella can be a helpful way to understand its essential role in breathing. Just as an umbrella expands and contracts, the diaphragm moves up and down with each breath, driving air in and out of the lungs.

This imagery highlights how the diaphragm facilitates full, efficient breathing, supporting oxygen intake and carbon dioxide release.

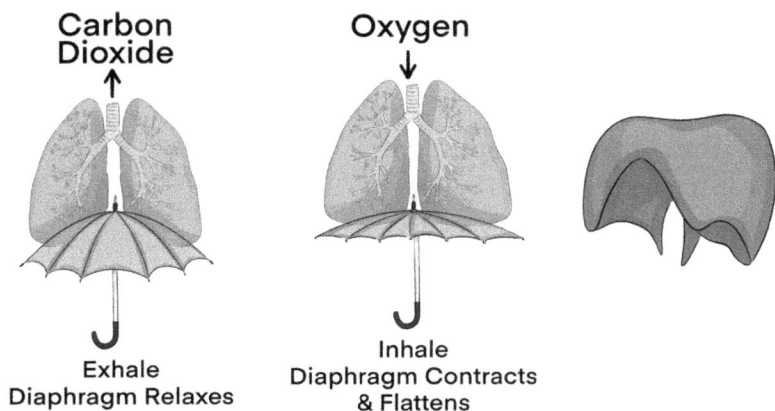

Carbon Dioxide ↑

Oxygen ↓

Exhale
Diaphragm Relaxes

Inhale
Diaphragm Contracts
& Flattens

Inhaling is an active process - As you breathe in, your diaphragm contracts, flattens, and moves downward, creating a vacuum (negative pressure) that pulls air into your lungs, making room for oxygen to fill them.

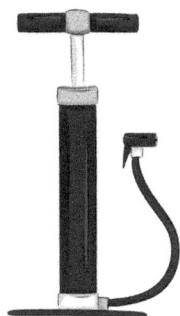

Think of it like using a bicycle pump: if you only raise the handle a little, you bring in just a small amount of air, meaning you'll need more pumps to fill the tire. But if you pull the handle all the way up, you bring in more air, filling the tire faster and with fewer pumps.

Exhaling is primarily a relaxed, passive process. When you breathe out, your diaphragm and rib muscles relax, shrinking the space in your chest cavity. This allows your lungs to deflate, gently pushing air out—like air escaping from a balloon. The natural elastic recoil of your lungs helps release the air without much effort. However, during forced exhalation—like blowing out a candle or during intense exercise—your abdominal and internal intercostal muscles kick in to push the air out more forcefully.

FLEXIBLE RIBCAGE

Together with the diaphragm, the intercostal muscles between your ribs are the primary muscles used for breathing. The ribcage plays a crucial role in both expanding and compressing the lungs during breathing, acting like a flexible framework to adjust the volume of the chest cavity.

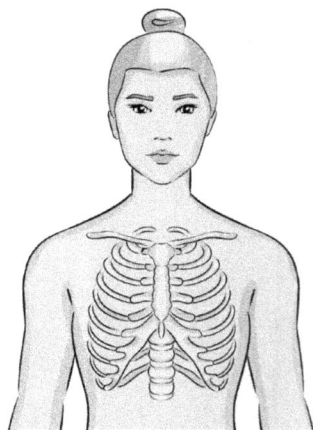

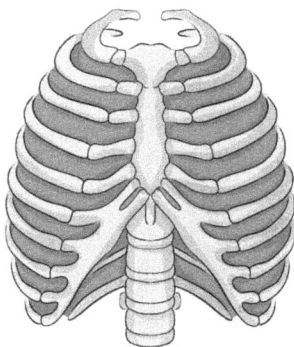

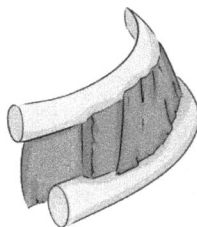

When you inhale, the diaphragm moves downward, and the external intercostals lift and expand the ribcage, allowing more air into the lungs. When you take a deep breath, you'll feel your ribcage expanding—not just top to bottom but also wide to the sides, to the front, and into your back. Your sternum (breastbone) also lifts slightly, increasing the front-to-back space.

When you exhale, your diaphragm and intercostal muscles relax, and the ribs move downward and inward, compressing the chest cavity and expelling air from the lungs.

WHERE THE VITAL EXCHANGE OF GAS TAKES PLACE – THE LUNGS

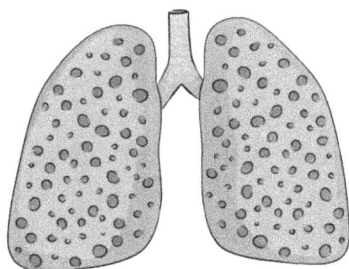

Your lungs sit protected within the ribcage, positioned above the diaphragm and on either side of the heart. They share the chest cavity with major blood vessels, such as the aorta and pulmonary arteries, which support oxygen and blood circulation. Since the heart and other organs take up space in the front, the lungs occupy more room in the back. [46] The lungs extend just above the collarbones from the front, reach about halfway down the ribcage, and expand toward the sides and back when fully inflated, ending just above the last rib.

As you inhale, oxygen travels down your windpipe, which splits into two bronchi—one for each lung, then into smaller bronchioles—ending in tiny, grape-like clusters called alveoli. These elastic alveoli stretch with each breath in and spring back when you exhale. Although each alveolus is tiny, there are around 480 million [47] of them, covering a surface area roughly the size of a tennis court. [48]

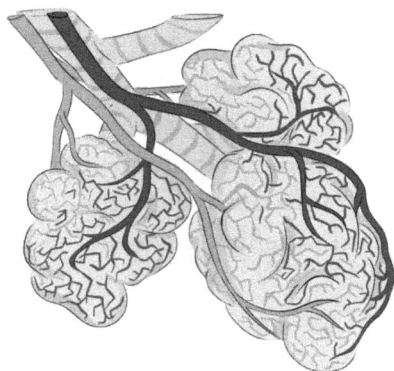

The alveoli are surrounded by tiny blood vessels called capillaries, where the crucial gas exchange so essential for life takes place. Red blood cells pick up oxygen from the lungs and deliver it throughout the body while simultaneously carrying carbon dioxide back to the lungs to be exhaled. When you exhale, the alveoli deflate, and carbon dioxide exits through your nose or mouth.

Since the lungs are wider at the bottom than the top, the inhaled oxygen needs to reach the lower part of the lungs, where the majority of air sacs (alveoli) and blood vessels are located. Most of the oxygen exchange occurs in these lower regions, making it essential for breathing techniques to focus on engaging the diaphragm to direct air deep into the lungs.

IMPROVE YOUR POSTURE - IMPROVE YOUR BREATHING

Your posture greatly affects the diaphragm's range of motion and how much air you can inhale. Since the diaphragm attaches to the ribs and spine, its movement during breathing also impacts digestion, elimination, and posture. Poor posture—

such as slumping, leaning forward, being overly rigid, collapsing, or habitually shifting weight to one leg—can restrict your diaphragm's motion.

Try sitting down and bending forward, then take a deep breath— it's hard, right? That's because your posture limits how well your diaphragm can move. Wearing tight clothing can have a similar effect, restricting the diaphragm and making it harder to breathe fully and comfortably.

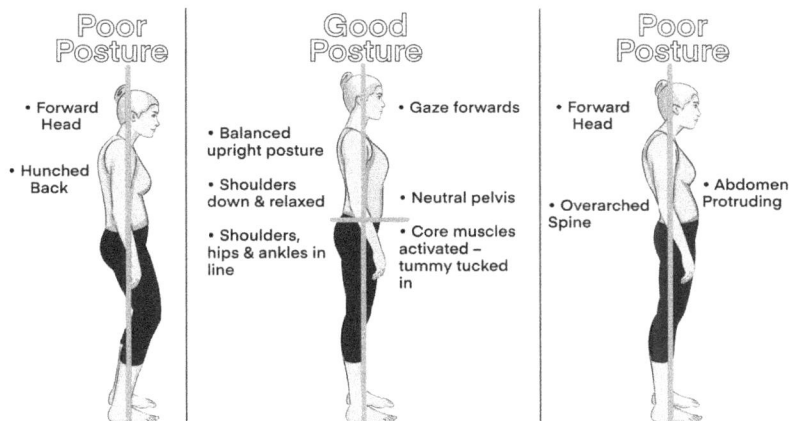

Poor Posture
- Forward Head
- Hunched Back

Good Posture
- Balanced upright posture
- Shoulders down & relaxed
- Shoulders, hips & ankles in line
- Gaze forwards
- Neutral pelvis
- Core muscles activated – tummy tucked in

Poor Posture
- Forward Head
- Overarched Spine
- Abdomen Protruding

Good posture means keeping a relaxed, upright position with your body aligned from head to feet. Your ears should align with your shoulders, shoulders with your hips, and hips over your ankles. Both feet should be evenly weighted on the ground and point forward, not outward.

When sitting, keep both feet flat on the floor (avoid crossing your legs). Sit upright with your shoulders aligned, engage your core, and distribute your weight evenly across both hips (without leaning). Picture your head balanced on your spine, like a golf ball on a tee, and avoid pushing it forward to see the screen. Also, avoid slouching or looking down at a screen for long periods, as this limits breathing and causes neck and eye strain. Adjust your screen so you can look straight ahead, maintaining a neutral posture.

You'll notice your posture improves as you practice the Five Tibetan Rites. Over time, staying upright will feel more natural, and maintaining alignment will become effortless.

Okay, let's begin!

EXPERIENCING WHERE THE BREATH MOVES IN YOUR BODY

If you have never experienced optimal depth, balance, and ease of breathing, how will you know whether you have it or not? [49]

—**Michael Grant White,** Optimal Breathing.

The first step is to learn how breathing affects the different spaces in your body involved in respiration. This exercise gives you a physical sensation of how these body parts move when you breathe in and out. They are not breathing techniques – just explorations of movement to help you improve your breathing.

Due to muscle tension and habitual breathing patterns, you may not experience the full range, depth, and volume of breathing described in the practices below. That's okay—just do the exercises as best as you can.

First, you will carry out a breathing exploration exercise for each of the following, and then you will combine them into one complete, fulfilling breath.

Note: *: Avoid deep forceful breathing and focus on a gentle, calmer, controlled breath throughout these exercises.*

> **TIP:** *Writing down your experiences after each exercise can be helpful. It provides a record to compare to later as you continue to practice and improve your breathing with the Rites.*

1. **Belly Breathing**
2. **Rib – Middle Chest Breathing**
3. **Collarbone – Upper Chest Breathing**
4. **Putting It All Together – One Complete Natural Breath**

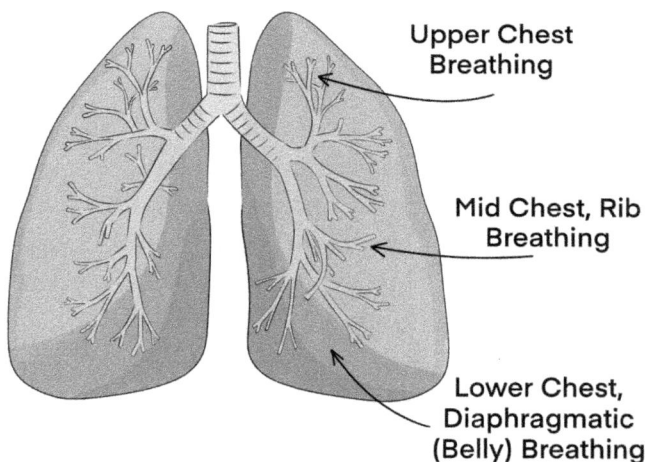

Upper Chest Breathing

Mid Chest, Rib Breathing

Lower Chest, Diaphragmatic (Belly) Breathing

What You Will Need For These Exercises

1. Loose, comfortable clothing so your breathing isn't restricted.

2. Use a scarf about the thickness of a silk one, with a mid-length—not too short or too long. If you don't have a scarf, a dressing gown sash, or a soft, flexible belt, it will work just as well. You will be lying on the ground, so make sure you are comfortable.

3. Support your head with a folded towel or low, firm pillow—but only so high that if you were standing, your head would be balanced on top of your spine (not tilted forward or backward).

BELLY (DIAPHRAGMATIC) BREATHING

Belly breathing, or diaphragmatic breathing, enables you to get the most air into your lungs. The lower part of your lungs rests on your diaphragm at the base of your ribcage. When you inhale, the diaphragm flattens and moves downward, drawing air into your lungs. As it lowers, it presses against your stomach, causing your belly to expand—hence the term "belly breathing." The more your stomach can expand with each inhale and contract with each exhale, the more effectively your diaphragm draws in oxygen and expels waste.

It's easier to practice this exercise lying down, as your stomach is more likely to relax in this position. Many people carry tension in their bellies, which can restrict diaphragm movement. Restoring its full range of motion may take time, so be patient with yourself. In the meantime, don't force your breathing—let it happen naturally and focus on gentle, gradual progress.

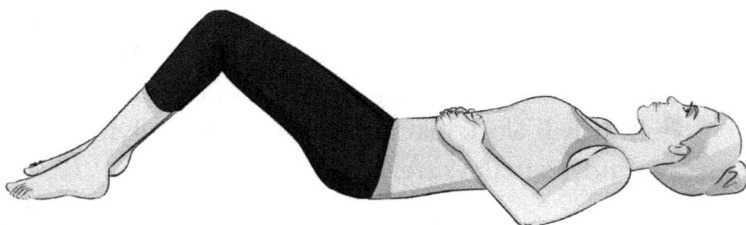

Aim: *To help you experience the effects of your belly swelling outwards when you inhale and retracting back towards your spine when you exhale.*

EXERCISE

- Place your hands over your belly button, with your fingertips slightly apart and loosely interlaced at the tips. Your fingertips (not fingers) will move apart on the in-breath and come back together on the out-breath.

- Allow your body and mind to relax for a few moments, as this will reduce tension in your breathing.

- When you are ready, take a normal breath in through your nose without hurrying—then exhale fully before breathing in.

- Inhale slowly through your nose. Your diaphragm will descend, pressing against the contents of your abdomen, which will expand outwards—spreading your fingertips slightly apart.

- Exhale slowly through your nose. Your diaphragm will relax and rise, and your stomach will flatten back towards your spine—bringing your fingertips inwards.

- Ensure you are not pulling your stomach in or pushing it out: allow the diaphragm's upward and downward (contract/relax) movement to do this unaided.

- Repeat several times until you can do this confidently.

RIB – MIDDLE CHEST BREATHING

Rib breathing uses the muscles between the ribs (the intercostals). During a full diaphragmatic breath, the rib cage lifts upward and spreads outwards (frontwards, sidewards, and backward) on inhalation. On exhalation, it collapses inward and down. The extent of this movement depends on the flexibility and strength of the intercostals and the diaphragm. Like other muscles, the intercostals can be strengthened and made more flexible through regular use, stretching, and breathing exercises.

You will need your scarf, dressing gown sash, or soft belt for this exercise.

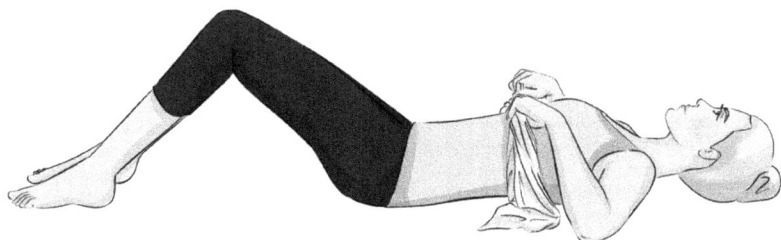

Aim: *To help you experience the sensation of your ribcage expanding outward on inhalation and collapsing inward on exhalation. The scarf provides resistance, making it easier to feel the extent of your ribcage's expansion and contraction.*

EXERCISE – Rib Breathing

- Spread out your scarf or sash so it lies flat behind your back around the lower third of your ribs, just under your breasts (or nipples for men). Hold each end loosely and lie down again.

- When lying down, cross one end of the scarf over the other in front of your chest in an X-shape, but don't tie the ends. Hold the material in each hand (as shown in the image above). You will pull the scarf firmly together as you exhale and allow it to slip through your fingers as the inhalation spreads it apart.

- Let the inhalation loosen the scarf so you can feel the strength of your breathing muscles expanding.

- During this exercise, you will continue to belly breathe, breathing slowly in and out through your nose. This time, the focus will be on the expansion and contraction of your ribcage.

- Begin to belly breathe as in the previous exercise. Once you are confidently and easily belly breathing, continue to do so throughout the exercise.

- Breathe out fully before inhaling, then exhale, pulling each end of the scarf together reasonably tightly. Then, breathe in, noticing how your ribs expand and press against the resistance of the scarf.

- Allow the scarf to slide slowly through your fingers as your ribcage lifts and expands outwards.

- Breathe out, noticing how your ribcage collapses inwards as you exhale—and progressively pull the scarf tighter as your ribcage returns to its normal size.

- Breathe in, expanding your ribs against the resistance of the scarf, and let the scarf slowly slide through your fingers as your ribs expand outwards.

- Breathe out, tightening the scarf as your ribcage collapses inwards. Try extending your exhalation by one or two seconds.

- Repeat this several times until you are confident with this step.

Rib Breathing On Its Own

The purpose of this exercise is to compare the fullness of diaphragmatic breathing with the limitations of rib breathing. Rib breathing alone is an incomplete form of breathing because it limits how much oxygen you take in. As a result, you may find yourself breathing more frequently with shallow, rapid breaths. This kind of breathing triggers the body's fight-or-flight response, leading to increased stress and anxiety over time.

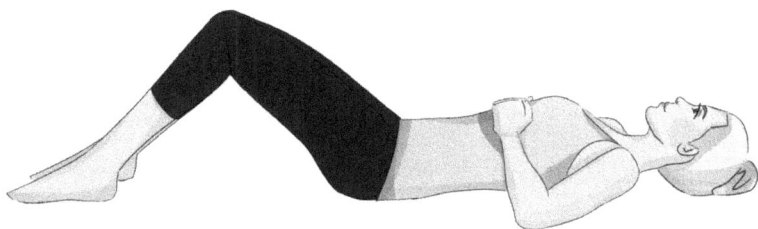

Aim: *To experience how your breathing capacity is reduced if you only breathe into your chest. Tightening your abdomen in this exercise restricts the downward movement of the diaphragm on inhalation, forcing the air higher into your chest.*

EXERCISE – Rib Breathing On Its Own

- Take a couple of normal breaths in through your nose without hurrying—then exhale fully before breathing in.
- Exhale, pulling your tummy inwards, and pulling each of the scarf ends together reasonably tightly.
- Keeping your belly pulled in, breathe into your mid-chest, allowing the scarf to slide progressively through your fingers as your ribcage expands.

- Breathe out and pull the scarf progressively tighter as your ribcage returns to its normal size.
- Observe how your breathing has become more rapid and shallow compared to belly breathing. Repeat this several times until you are confident with this step.

COLLARBONE - UPPER CHEST BREATHING

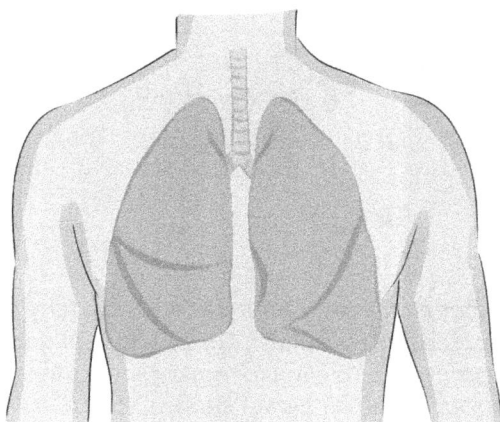

As you can see from the illustration above, the top of your lungs has the smallest area of volume. The highest point of your lungs lies just above your collarbones and then widens across your chest, armpits, and upper back. During relaxed breathing, you do not need to use the accessory breathing muscles in the shoulders, neck, and collarbone—they remain inactive unless you experience shortness of breath.

When the accessory breathing muscles activate, they lift the breastbone, ribs, and collarbones to create extra space for the lungs to expand. These muscles kick in to help with breathing during intense activity, blowing up a balloon, singing, low oxygen at high altitudes, or respiratory illnesses. However, they often get overused in day-to-day life—some people unnecessarily and unconsciously raise their shoulders when inhaling during normal activities.

The problem with relying too much on these upper chest muscles is that it can lead to tension and stiffness, making breathing feel more effortful. Plus, upper chest breathing is the least efficient—it takes a lot of energy for very little air, leaving you feeling tense, tired, and out of breath more easily.

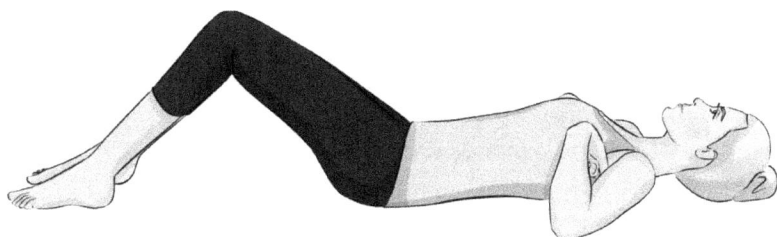

Aim: *To feel your breastbone lift and your ribcage expand upward and outward in your upper chest. Use your fists like you used the scarf earlier to create resistance, helping you better sense the expansion and contraction of your ribcage. The movement will be subtle—you might notice a slight lift in your shoulders or feel the upper back expanding as it presses lightly against the floor.*

EXERCISE – Upper Chest Breathing

- During this exercise, the focus will be on the expansion and contraction of your upper chest.

- Make loose fists with both hands and place them in the middle (or close to the middle) of your armpits (see illustration above). If this is uncomfortable, cross your arms and place the fingers of each hand in the middle of the opposite armpit.

- Begin to belly breathe. Once you are easily and confidently breathing in this manner, continue to do so throughout the exercise.

- Breathe out fully before inhaling, then exhale, pressing your fists firmly but lightly into your armpits.

- Then, breathe in. When your ribcage is fully expanded, inhale a bit more without overstraining, and allow the air to fill the upper part of your lungs. Notice the slight pressure pushing back against the top of your fingers as your ribcage expands and widens.

- Breathe out, observing how your ribcage lowers and collapses inwards as you exhale, relaxing the pressure of your fists as it does so.

- Try this a few times, noticing how your breastbone and upper chest are being drawn toward your head, rising with inhalation, and falling with exhalation. Don't lift your shoulders to achieve this—allow the inhalation to move the ribcage upward and outwards.

- Repeat several times until you are confident with this step.

A COMPLETE NATURAL BREATH

The final level is to combine these three steps to form one smooth, continuous, and wave-like movement—a complete natural breath. Your breathing spaces will fill with air like you are gently blowing up a balloon, from the belly to the ribs and into the upper chest—like a wave originating in the pelvis moving up the spine and ending at the nose as you breathe out.

Although belly breathing is a good start in learning to breathe deeply, your breathing is a *round* movement. A true deep breath expands the body in a 360-degree radius. The belly swells with the downward motion of the diaphragm and remains extended as the ribcage widens and lifts, expanding air into the sides of your body and into the back.

"Most of the lung volume is actually contained in the back of the body. The belly only comprises about 40% of the total breathing volume. Breathing into the belly will steer the person in a better direction than focusing on the upper chest, but true deep breathing does not end there." [50]

—**Michael Grant White,** Optimal Breathing.

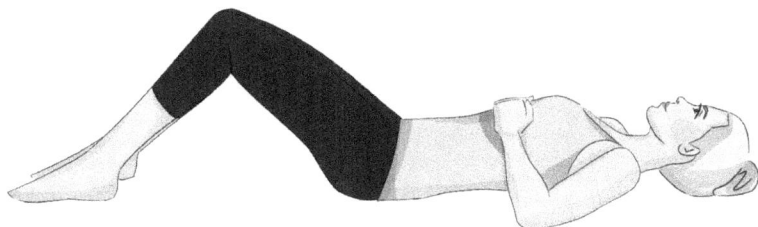

EXERCISE

- Place your hands on your upper belly—fingers tips lightly interlinked and touching. As you inhale, your fingertips will move slightly part, and as you exhale, your fingertips will come together.

- Take a couple of normal breaths, then exhale fully.

- In a continuous, smooth, and easy movement, breathe in slowly through your nose, expanding your abdomen, then your ribcage (to the front, sides, and back), and finally your upper chest.

- Breathe out slowly and smoothly—as your abdomen flattens back toward your spine, your ribs lower and collapse inward, and your upper chest lowers and retracts inward.

- Try this a couple of times until you are confident with the movement.

PART TWO

THE BREATHING EXERCISES WITH THE RITES

8

HOW TO PRACTICE THE BREATHING EXERCISES WITH THE RITES

1. "Energy Breathing"
2. How to Breath When Practicing The Rites.

ENERGY BREATHING

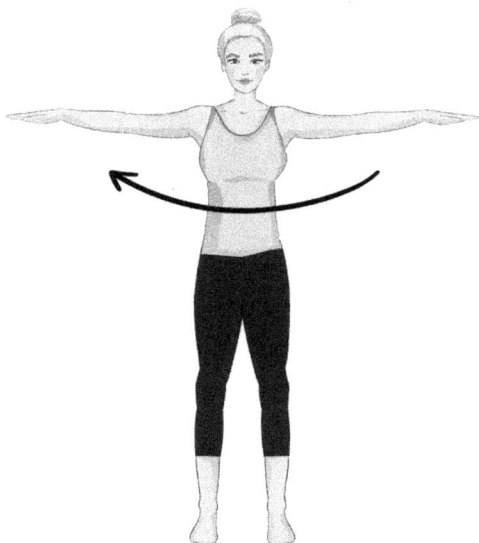

Tibetan Rite No. 1 – The Spin

You are now ready to learn T5T's Energy Breathing Exercise—the three "Energy Breaths" that are carried out between each Rite. The goal is to promote natural, full breathing, expanding and strengthening your respiratory capacity. With regular practice, your everyday breathing will improve.

You have already learned the importance of breathing through your nose, strengthening your diaphragm by using it as your primary breathing muscle—and enhancing the strength and flexibility of your ribcage and your entire breathing apparatus from your pelvis to your nose. You have also learned how the breath moves in the breathing spaces of your body—and have experienced your breath as a round and full movement. Now, the focus is on deep, steady breathing with minimal effort, helping you feel more energized, calm, and replenished.

You will carry out these three deep Energy Breaths between each Rite to help improve your stamina, boost your energy, and reduce stress. I call it Energy Breathing because it reduces fatigue, lifts your spirits, restores calm, and improves well-being. The energy I am referring to is not a caffeine-like instant high that exhausts quickly but a calm, sustaining, enduring energy. The former type of energy burns you out, while Energy Breathing replenishes you.

Energy Breathing aims to remove the tensions in your breathing to achieve natural full breathing, where your body's respiratory muscles function optimally. With time and practice, your breathing will become more elastic and mobile. As you learn to breathe more fully and deeply, you will experience a new awakening of energy and enthusiasm for life.

Energy Breathing is yoga for the breath. Its purpose is to –

- Gently stretch, strengthen, open, and expand all your respiratory muscles.

- The long, slow exhalation is intended to calm and de-stress you as it stimulates your parasympathetic nervous system.

- Allowing a natural pause after exhalation, followed by an effortless inhalation, encourages slower, more mindful breathing. In today's fast-paced world, many people rush from one task to the next, leaving little room for pauses. This constant focus on the future can cause us to lose touch with the present moment.

- This daily reminder of your breathing helps you become more aware of your daily breathing patterns. You will notice when you are restricting the full potential of your breathing and will become alert to the particular situations that trigger this response. By changing your breathing, you can adjust your reaction.

When you practice energy Breathing with real awareness in the present moment, it is wonderfully fulfilling and very calming. When you have mastered it, it is smooth and even and fills you up without any strain at all. You can feel the breath massage your spine and organs as it rolls up and down your body. The exhalation is a marvelous opportunity to "let go" in the largest sense of the word; and the inhalation allows something new and fresh to come in.

It really is possible to change the way you *live* your life by the way you *breathe* your life.

Breathe deeply and gently through every cell of the body, laugh happily, and release the head of all worries and anxieties; and finally, breathe in the blessing of love and hope that is flowing in the air; and you will understand the meaning of the human breath.

—**Pundit Acharya,** Indian mystic and author of *Breath, Sleep, the Heart, and Life*

ENERGY BREATHING AND THE COMPLETE YOGIC BREATH

T5T's Energy Breathing method is my adapted version of the well-known yogic breathing technique called the *3-Part Breath* or the *Complete Yogic Breath,* a foundational practice used by many practitioners, not just during yoga practices.

If you already know how to do the Complete Yogic Breath— Energy Breathing has adaptations and a specific focus—to remove tension from our breathing apparatus and to open our breathing spaces on a daily basis. These adaptations include the following:

- Begins with an exhalation
- Lengthens the exhalation
- Rests in the pause before the in-breath
- Allows the inhalation to arrive by itself without forcing or rushing it
- Adds affirmations, visualizations, and mantras

Note for Yoga Practitioners: The Complete Yogic Breath is taught differently from teacher to teacher and often includes the instructions to exhale in the reverse order to that in which you inhaled.

Inhale. Belly – Ribs – Upper Chest.

Exhale. Upper Chest – Ribs – Belly.

In Energy Breathing, you exhale in the same sequence as you inhale—inhalation and exhalation follow the same pattern: belly, ribs, and upper chest.

LET'S BEGIN

Control the breath carefully. Inhalation gives strength and a controlled body; retention gives steadiness of mind and longevity; exhalation purifies body and spirit.

—Goraksasatakam,
early Hatha yoga text from the 11th-12th century

You may recall from What Happens When We Breathe in Chapter 2, that your brain primarily regulates breathing in response to high carbon dioxide levels rather than oxygen levels in your blood—unless the oxygen levels drop significantly, as they might at high altitudes or with certain respiratory diseases. When CO_2 levels rise in the blood, the brain signals the diaphragm and other respiratory muscles to contract, prompting you to inhale.

Energy Breathing follows this entirely natural respiratory pattern. First, you will exhale, allow a natural pause, and then inhale. The exhalation triggers the next inhale, as rising CO_2 levels prompt your brain to signal the diaphragm to contract, initiating the breath. This sequence—exhale, pause, inhale—is the foundation of T5T's Energy Breathing practice.

1. Exhalation
2. Pause
3. Inhalation

1. Exhalation

Unless you breathe out fully, you cannot breathe in completely. For example, If you fill an already half-filled cup, you are only topping it up, not filling it up completely. If you extend your exhalation to its full conclusion, a deeper inhalation will occur naturally, and more oxygen will be available to your lungs. You can never empty your lungs totally, for a portion of air will remain in your lungs to keep them from collapsing. [51]

Exhalation is a passive release of the tension created during inhalation, requiring no active muscle use. It is usually followed by a natural pause (although dysfunctional breathing patterns can disrupt this). Lengthening your exhalation enhances relaxation, and extending the pause deepens that sense of calm and letting go of tension. This slower, steady breathing slows your breathing rate, promotes deeper inhalation, and allows more time for oxygen to transfer from the lungs into the bloodstream.

You are trying too hard if you find yourself suddenly grabbing for air. Instead, let your exhalation lengthen naturally, without any strain. Don't prolong your exhalation beyond what is comfortable; concentrate on slowing the air leaving your body. Long exhalations are calming. They are intuitively a time to let go and release. As you breathe out, let all your muscles relax—feel the tension leaving your body.

2. Pause

Between the end of a natural exhalation and the start of a new inhalation, the breath naturally pauses for around 1-2 seconds. This moment offers a sense of calm and stillness, allowing the body's muscles and nervous system to reset before the next breath. Some describe this pause as a rare experience of true presence. However, many people, accustomed to rushing or anxious and stressed by daily life, either skip these pauses by grabbing for air or breathing rapidly and shallowly, missing out on this natural moment of peace.

Here's how to encourage a longer, comfortable pause and apply it to your Energy Breathing exercise.

- Sit upright on a straight-backed chair and relax for a few natural breaths.
- Wait until you feel relaxed, then breathe out slowly.
- At the end of the exhalation, relax in the pause for as long as it is comfortable—and then let your inhalation arise naturally by itself. Sometimes, it will feel like your in-breath has come from a long way away—almost as if you are being breathed.

Since the brain primarily regulates breathing based on carbon dioxide levels, when people chronically over-breathe, such as during anxious states, CO_2 levels drop, disturbing the body's normal, natural drive to pause between breaths. For people who struggle to achieve these natural pauses, practicing diaphragmatic breathing regularly, as you shall during Energy Breathing, can help re-establish balance and calm the nervous system.

3. Inhalation

The inhalation process begins with the diaphragm contracting and moving downward. As you breathe in, the diaphragm pushes against the contents of your abdomen, causing your belly to expand outward. Simultaneously, your ribcage lifts and widens, creating space for the lungs to fill. Think of it like inflating a balloon—not only does the air expand forward into the belly and chest, but it also spreads outward in all directions: to the sides, front, and back—a 360-degree movement—not just up and down as some mistakenly believe.

> *Remember, your breathing is a ROUND movement. The lungs inflate like a balloon inside the ribcage, expanding in all directions: to the front, to the back, around the sides, and up and down.*

Here are some essential points to remember before you start learning the exercises.

Never Suppress Your Body's Natural Urges

Never suppress your body's natural urges—if you need to take a short breath, do so. Avoid overdoing your breathing, especially by inhaling forcefully or taking rapid breaths in quick succession. Focus on a gentle, calmer, controlled breath throughout these exercises. Gradually lengthen your exhalations, which will slow your breathing and help restore a sense of calm.

Breathe Only Through The Nose

When you practice The Five Tibetan Rites, breathe only through your nose. Breathing through your nose slows the airflow into your lungs, giving more time for oxygen to be absorbed into your bloodstream. Nasal breathing also filters, warms, and humidifies the air.

Don't Rush Through Your Three Energy Breaths

During your T5T practice, don't rush through your three Energy Breaths between each Rite. Rushing can turn an enjoyable and beneficial activity into yet another task. The breathing exercises should not be merely mechanical—keep your awareness entirely focused on your breathing as you are doing it. You won't be present if you are hurrying.

Practice In A Pollution-Free Environment

Since deeper breathing draws air deep into your lungs, it's important to ensure the air is as clean as possible. Avoid burning incense or candles, which can release irritants and pollutants into the air. Additionally, try to avoid extreme temperatures—both hot and cold air as they can irritate the respiratory system and make breathing less comfortable.

Slow and Quiet – Steady and Even

Aim for your breathing to be slow, quiet, and consistent without changes in volume. A loud breath can indicate unnecessary strain. Focus on keeping each breath smooth, steady, and even, gradually eliminating any jerks or pauses. As you relax into this rhythm, allow the sense of deep calm from your breathing to take hold and settle within you.

Easy, No Forcing or Pushing

Energy Breathing should always be gentle and relaxed. Avoid filling your lungs to maximum capacity since this can create stiffness and strain. Instead, aim for around 80% capacity or less, breathing slowly and getting familiar with your limits. Never push or force your breathing. When you breathe out, empty your lungs to about 30% of your capacity and pause for a second or two before breathing in again. You'll enjoy the experience more if you don't try too hard – Energy Breathing should not be an effort. The goal is to keep it effortless and enjoyable. If you find yourself gasping for air, it's a sign you're trying too hard and need to ease up.

Never Pull Your Belly Inwards To Exhale

Keep your belly relaxed and focus on slowing the out-breath. This activates the parasympathetic nervous system, promoting the rest-and-digest response, which helps reduce stress and improve mental clarity. Pulling your belly in during inhalation restricts the diaphragm's movement, limiting how much it can descend and reducing the amount of oxygen you can take in.

ENERGY BREATHING STEPS: ONE, TWO, AND THREE

In *The Eye of Revelation,* Colonel Bradford explains that for the Rites to work most effectively, we need to build up to twenty-one repetitions of each of the Five Rites. This is achieved by practicing just three repetitions in your first week, then adding two additional repetitions each week until you are doing the full twenty-one repetitions in ten weeks' time.

Adding Energy Breathing to the Rites works like this.

- Week 1 – **Energy Breathing (Step One)** - when doing 3 repetitions of each Rite.
- Week 2 – **Energy Breathing (Step Two)** – when doing 5 repetitions of each Rite.
- Week 3 - **Energy Breathing (Step Three)** – when doing 7 repetitions of each Rite.
- Weeks 4 -10 – You will continue to use **Energy Breathing, Step Three.**

Already Practicing The Rites?

If you are already practicing the Rites and want to add Energy Breathing—do Step One for a week, Step Two for the next week, and Step Three during your third week of practice. Continue indefinitely with Energy Breathing, Step Three, for as long as you practice the Rites—and if not, as a practice in its own right. **Note:** Since Energy Breathing is carried out in the same position as you finish each Rite, refer to the instructions in Part Three.

What You Need to Begin

Begin by lying on your back on the floor. For added comfort, place a blanket beneath you. Use a small pillow or folded towel under your head and neck to keep your chin in a neutral position—not tilted too far forward or backward. This ensures your throat remains relaxed and strain-free, optimizing your breathing.

STEP ONE, ENERGY BREATHING

Remain at this level for WEEK ONE of your practice.

Place your hands on your ribs just under your breastbone, with the tips of your fingers interlaced and touching in the middle (the Energy Breathing Position.) You will be able to feel the expansion of your belly with your lower fingers and the expansion of your ribs with your upper fingers. As you breathe in, your fingertips will part; as you breathe out, they will come together again—this is not a big movement.

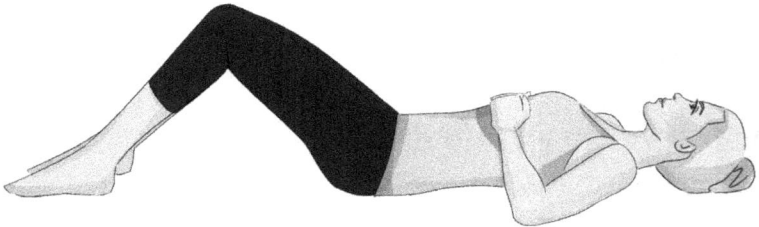

- Place your hands in the Energy Breathing Position. (See image above.)
- Close your eyes so you can tune in to your breathing.
- Relax your eyes, face, and jaw.
- Exhale fully through your nose to begin and continue to breathe through your nose throughout Energy Breathing.

- Breathe in, expanding your abdomen, then your rib cage, and finally, the upper portion of your lungs, just under your collarbones. Breathe out slowly in the same manner, flattening your abdomen, then contracting your ribs and lowering your ribcage.
- Work toward gradually slowing your exhalation to about twice the length of your inhalation.
- Wait in the pause for as long as is comfortable until the new and fuller inhalation arrives naturally.
- Carry out two more extended exhalations, finishing with an inhalation.

STEP TWO, ENERGY BREATHING WITH ADDED AFFIRMATION

Remain at this level for the SECOND WEEK of your practice.

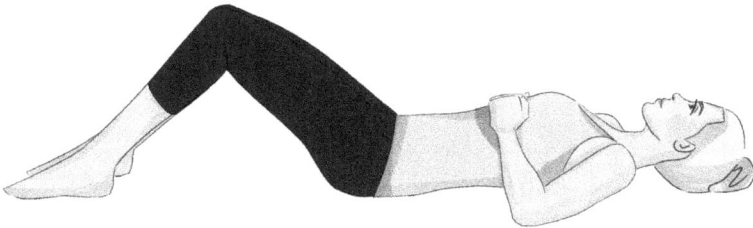

Step two is the same as Step one, with the following additional steps:

During the exhalation

- As you exhale, let the muscles in your neck, shoulders, chest, arms, and stomach go limp, relaxing your body as you do so.
- Allow your body weight to sink deeply into the earth below.
- As you breathe out, imagine you are letting go of all the tension and problems of your day. Say silently to yourself, **"LET GO."**

During the pause

- Focus on relaxing any areas where you feel tension.

During the inhalation

- Due to the extended exhalation and pause before each subsequent inhalation, your in-breaths will require less effort.
- Remember to relax your stomach and allow the new inhalation to flow in slowly through your nose. Say silently to yourself, **"THIS IS FOR ME."**

STEP THREE, ENERGY BREATHING WITH SACRED MANTRA

Commence this final level during the THIRD WEEK of your practice.

Step three is the same as Steps One and Two but includes a special mantra to help calm and focus your mind so you can enjoy every moment of your Five Tibetans practice. Then, having completed your daily practice, you can take the new energy, focus, and calm you gained into your everyday life.

A mantra is a tool to develop concentration. *"SO HUM"* is a sacred mantra that reinforces the natural sound of breathing and means, "That I Am" or "I Am That."

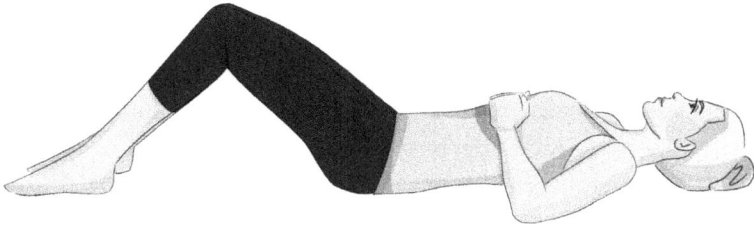

- When you breathe in, imagine you are drawing the breath up through your feet, and as you do so, say, **"SO"** silently to yourself. Observe the natural opening and expansion of your breathing spaces.

- When you breathe out, imagine the breath leaving through the crown of your head and say **"HUM"** silently to yourself. Notice how this seems to squeeze even the deepest air out of your lungs.

HOW TO BREATHE WHEN PRACTICING THE FIVE TIBETAN RITES

The aim is to energize each Rite with a steady, rhythmic breathing pattern that maximizes oxygen uptake without adding tension.

During exercise, your body needs more oxygen to fuel muscles and releases more carbon dioxide. As a result, breathing during these exercises becomes stronger and deeper in contrast to the gentler, slower breathing used in Energy Breathing.

The Breathing Method While Practicing the Rites

The Five Tibetan Rites (except the first one) consist of two parts.

- The **First Part:** Begins in the starting position and moves "up" or "into" the peak of the movement.
- The **Second Part:** Moves "down" "or back" from the peak to the original starting position.

How to incorporate your breathing with each of the Five Tibetan Rites

1. *Breathe in all the way up*—into the first part of the posture
2. *Breathe out all the way down*— into the second part of the posture

When performed correctly, each movement flows naturally with the breath: one inhalation powers the entire first part of the movement, and one exhalation carries you through the second part. This creates a continuous, smooth rhythm, aligning breath and movement seamlessly.

The exception to this breathing pattern is the 1ˢᵗ Rite, which is one continuous movement— spinning around with your arms outstretched. Many people unconsciously hold their breath while concentrating, a habit common in daily life and during exercises. To avoid this, take a breath before you start spinning and remind yourself to keep breathing throughout the movement.

Nose Breathing Is More Efficient Than Mouth Breathing

Researchers from the University of Western Australia, Perth, compared mouth and nose breathing during exercise and concluded that nose breathing is more efficient than mouth breathing regarding oxygen uptake.[52] When carrying out the Rites, continue breathing through your nose to improve diaphragmatic strength and flexibility through nasal resistance while also maximizing oxygen uptake.

MONITORING YOUR BREATHING WHILE PRACTICING THE RITES

When practicing the Rites, your breathing should be slow, full, and quiet—a fulfilling, nourishing, and replenishing breath, not loud or forced with harsh sniffing sounds through the nose. As your repetitions increase, your body will naturally need more oxygen, and your breathing may deepen and become more frequent. This will vary from person to person, depending on their fitness level.

Monitoring your breathing while doing the Rites helps you stay in tune with your body. If your breathing becomes loud, erratic, or strained, it may be a sign that you're pushing too hard. Avoid holding your breath or forgetting to breathe, as it reduces your oxygen uptake and energy levels.

Aim for your breathing to be smooth, steady, and even. Focus on the smoothness and evenness of your breath, gradually eliminating jerks and pauses. Synchronize your breathing with the movements with your movements—merging breath and motion into one seamless flowing experience. If you need to take another breath, do so—as your breathing will gradually become more extended and deeper with practice, and eventually, you will be able to synchronize the length of your breathing with the length of your movement—breathing and movement as one.

FURTHER TIPS TO IMPROVE YOUR BREATHING

1. **Practice the Five Tibetan Rites!** This popular daily routine improves both flexibility and strength. It stretches and strengthens your body in almost every direction, expanding your range of motion and helping you breathe more fully and with less effort. It improves flexibility, helping relieve tension in overused muscles in the neck, shoulders, hips, and back. It strengthens muscles that have become weak from underuse and helps adjust muscle imbalances—strong on one side, weak on another. It helps improve your posture by strengthening the muscles that support you in remaining in an aligned upright position instead of slumped or slouched over. It relieves stiffness and increases energy so you can do more and be more. Coupled with the breathing improvement practices outlined in this book, you have a go-anywhere, do-at-anytime exercise routine that takes only a short amount of time per day for such great benefits.

2. **Enjoy Being More Active.** Your daily Five Tibetan Rites practice will give you more energy and motivation.

Try incorporating activities that also stretch and strengthen your body and help improve your breathing in the process, like swimming or rowing (on the water or using the rowing machine) or any activity that gets you moving and enjoying life. Spend more time outside enjoying nature and hopefully the fresh air where you live.

3. **Practice Good Posture – Standing, Sitting, Or Lying.** Good posture is integral to good breathing. It maximizes the ability of your breathing spaces to open fully allowing you to obtain vital oxygen without straining to do so. A crunched-over body does the opposite—it restricts your breathing. Refer to the instructions for good posture in Chapter 6 - Improve Your Posture - Improve Your Breathing, and when you are sitting, try this.

   - **Sitting**. Keep your back mostly upright with your natural curves intact (lumbar, thoracic, and cervical.) Keep your shoulders back but relaxed, and align your ears over your collarbones (avoid forward head posture or chin jutting). Have both feet resting flat on the floor, and keep your weight evenly balanced on both hips. Make sure your knees are even with your hips or slightly below. Look straight ahead, aligning your computer screen with your eyes so you don't need to lower your head. Keeping a heavy head upright all day when working causes neck strain.
   - **Your Sleeping Posture**. If you sleep on your side, try placing a pillow between your legs. The weight of one leg on top of the other is heavy, and the pillow absorbs some of that load. It also helps

keep your spine aligned and your airways open so you can breathe better. If you sleep on your back, try placing a pillow under your knees, but sleeping on your back is not recommended if you snore or have sleep apnea.

Sleeping on your side is generally the best position if you're a snorer. Sleeping on your back can cause the tongue and soft tissues in your throat to relax and fall backward, partially blocking the airway and increasing snoring. Side sleeping helps keep the airway open, reducing snoring and improving airflow throughout the night.

4. **Sing**. Consider taking singing lessons or joining classes or groups that practice singing. Practice singing in the shower or walking about—wherever it is private and you won't disturb people. Singing helps improve your breathing by strengthening your breathing muscles as well as your voice.

5. **Practice Using Diaphragmatic Breathing In Your Daily Life.** Now you have learned how to use your diaphragm when practicing the Rites, try using it during your daily activities, such as walking, in the shower, climbing stairs, sitting at your desk, in a social setting, and so on.

6. **The Air In Your Home**. Avoid breathing in lung irritants like artificial fragrances, mold, dust, smoking, or secondhand smoke. Check the labels on your candles and incense to avoid breathing toxic substances. Consider investing in air filters if you can afford them or feel they are necessary.

7. **Practice Mindfulness and Meditate Regularly.** It doesn't have to be complicated; just spend some time each day focusing on your breathing without trying to control it.

For further breathing resources, including books, apps, products, accessories, workshops, etc, please see Further Information at the back of this book.

9

BREATHING MEDITATIONS WITH THE RITES

In our modern world, there seems to be a never-ending need for things to move faster and faster toward some future event. We find it hard to relax and to experience the present moment. Finding time to experience the peace in silence has become something we must schedule into our lives. If you even remotely believe, as the ancients did, that we have only a finite number of breaths before we expire, then spending those breaths wisely will not only prolong your life but will also improve the quality of your life.

Often, people find they are making lists of things to do, people to call, stuff to buy, actions to take, and so on before and during their Five Tibetans practice. Sometimes, try as they might, people are often distracted and cannot be present in their mind and body. These first two meditation techniques focused on breathing are short but effective—they replace the stress response with the relaxation response. You can use them anytime, but they work well before starting your Five Tibetans practice, so you can focus on being here now.

The third meditation is when you have the time and desire to go deeper into a guided meditation. It works particularly well after you have completed your Rites practice, but you can also use it at any time.

You can also download the audio versions of these breathing meditations on my T5T.com website for free.

As for the proper inner breath, it is called the embryonic breath. Since it is naturally inside you, you do not have to see outside for it.

—Master Great Nothing of Sung-Shan,
from the Taoist Canon on Breathing

THE "BE HERE NOW" BREATHING TECHNIQUE

This short breathing meditation helps bring you into the present moment when the mind is distracted before practicing the Five Tibetan Rites—or at any time. One to two minutes is usually sufficient, but this technique can be extended for as long as you desire and can be used for meditation. Some practitioners call this technique the "One Minute Meditation" and use it frequently during stressful moments in their daily lives.

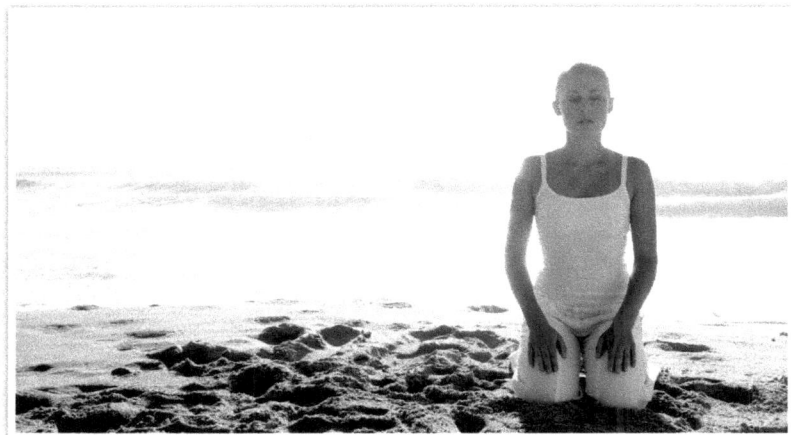

The best time to use this breathing technique is when your mind is preoccupied with other things. If you feel scattered and 'not present' when you do T5T, you may not be aware of when you are straining your body. The "Be Here Now" breathing technique helps combat the self-defeating and stress-inducing habit of rushing and will prevent your practice from becoming just another task to be completed.

INSTRUCTIONS

- Sit in a comfortable position with your hands resting in your lap, or lie on the floor with your knees bent and your hands resting by your sides so you don't restrict your breathing. Close your eyes.

- Breathing through your nose, begin by exhaling fully. Then, breathe in, take a slow, deep breath, and exhale slowly through your nose.

- Breathing normally, mentally scan your body from your toes to the top of your head, consciously relaxing your muscles deeply as you do so. Pay special attention to your jaw and hands, which typically hold lots of tension due to clenching.

- Become aware of your breathing.

- On your next exhalation, say silently to yourself, "Breathing Out." *Experience* yourself slowly breathing out.

- As you rest in the pause before the next in-breath, say silently to yourself, "Pause." *Experience* yourself pausing.

- As you breathe in, say silently to yourself, "Breathing In." *Experience* yourself breathing in.

- Continue in this manner, saying your breathing rhythm silently to yourself while you *experience* your breathing.

- *Breathing out*

- *Pause*

- *Breathing in*
- *Breathing out*
- *Pause*
- *Breathing in*
- Breathe easily and naturally in this manner for one to two minutes or until you feel calm and centered. If you find your mind wandering, don't worry; bring your awareness back to experiencing your breathing rhythm and silently say each step to yourself.
- When you are ready, open your eyes and allow your awareness to return to the room.

THE ONE BREATH

A short breathing meditation to help centre you before practicing the Rites, or at any time.

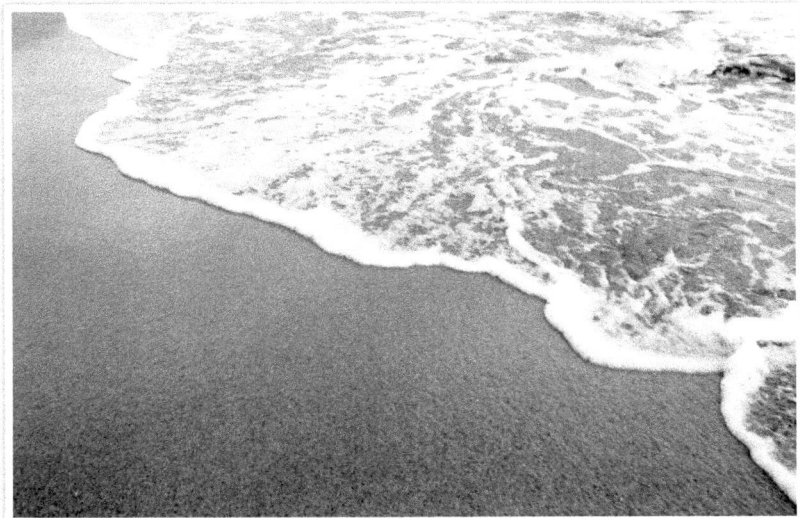

The One Breath is a simple and potentially profound relaxation and stress-management technique. It is a very useful exercise when you don't have much time and want to harmonize your mind, body, and spirit. It is also an excellent way to end your T5T practice, helping you establish a sense of peace for the remainder of your day. This exercise is equally effective for brief and extended periods, including meditation, and can also assist you in going to sleep.

Before you begin, consider this: the air on this planet is constantly recycled, and all living things share this air, breathing in nutrients and breathing out wastes. When we are born, we take our first breath of this communal earth air; when we die, we return our last breath to the earth. Keeping this awareness in mind before you begin this exercise can help you relax and trust your breath more deeply.

While you sleep, your breathing is automatic, almost as if "you are being breathed." During this exercise, you will become conscious of the breath, but you will also try to maintain the perception that *you have to do nothing except allow yourself to be breathed.*

Your aims

To initiate the relaxation response and to experience the fullness of your breath without the usual day-to-day restrictions.

INSTRUCTIONS

- Sit or lie in a comfortable position with your eyes closed.

- Breathe through your nose throughout the exercise.

- Bring your attention to your breathing and just observe it without trying to control it in any way.

- Now relax further and simply observe (witness) the natural ebb and flow of the breath being breathed into you and then withdrawn from you. Notice how and where the breath moves you: how your spine lowers and lifts and how your head rolls slightly forward and backward.

- As you feel the breath being breathed into you, imagine this life-enhancing breath entering your body and permeating every single cell, from the tips of your toes to the tip of your nose.

- As you exhale, imagine all the waste gases from your cells flowing toward your lungs and leaving with each breath.

- Surrender yourself to the feeling of being breathed for a few minutes. If your mind wanders, simply bring your awareness back to this exercise and continue.

- Notice how your breathing has slowed and deepened as you no longer attempt to control it. It is almost as if a deep, slow, natural breath has always been with you.

- When you are ready, begin to breathe normally once more. Allow yourself a few moments to reorient yourself before getting up and moving, calm and alert, into your day.

THE ENERGISING HEALING BREATH

If you have time after your Five Tibetan Rites practice, this fifteen-minute breathing meditation is a wonderful way to maximize your benefits.

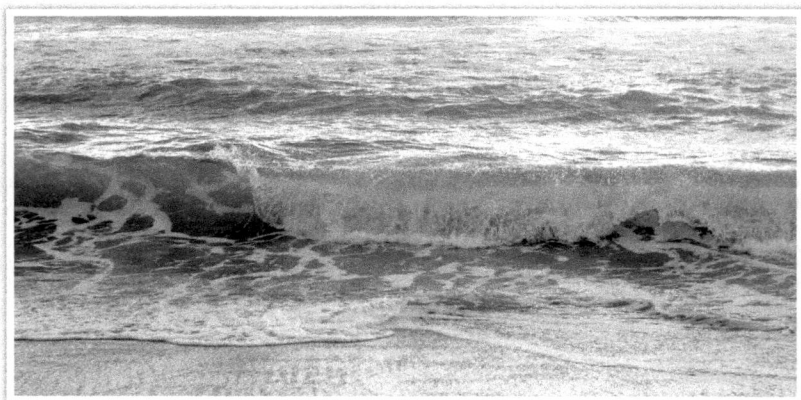

This final meditation is perfect for those who wish to perform a deeper healing and reenergizing of their body. It is beneficial after completing your Five Tibetans practice, during which you can focus on those areas that felt stiff, tense, weak, or imbalanced as you carried out the Rites – and release them. It utilizes the power of visualization to assist in healing these "stuck" areas and provides a wonderful feeling of well-being and calm that will last throughout your day.

It can be practiced for extended periods as a relaxation or stress-control technique or to assist you in falling asleep.

You can download this meditation (and the two above) for free on my T5T.com website or memorize the simple instructions below.

Your aims

To utilize the power of visualization to rejuvenate and enrich your body with nutrient-rich oxygen and life energy (*prana*)— and to remove wastes. To relax, restoring new energy and vitality to your body, mind, and soul.

INSTRUCTIONS

- Lie or sit comfortably so no aches or discomfort will disturb your attention. If lying, have your knees bent with your feet on the floor and your arms by your sides. If sitting, have your legs slightly apart and your arms resting in your lap.

- Relax, and allow your weight to surrender you to the floor or the chair. If sitting, ensure your back is straight, and your shoulders are relaxed.

- Close your eyes, relax your face and jaw, and begin to breathe in and out through your nose. Focus your awareness on the gentle ebb and flow of your breathing.

- Now, begin to double or simply extend your exhalation. Establish the rhythm of breath that is most fluid, smooth, and relaxing for your body while continuing to double or extend your exhalation time.

- As you inhale, visualize fresh oxygen moving throughout your body, energizing each and every cell. As you exhale, visualize the carbon dioxide and other wastes moving out of your body.

- Bring your attention to your nose, where the air is entering your body. Imagine the oxygen and life force swirling through your nasal passages and throat and down into and around your lungs. Tell yourself that with every breath you take in, healing energy is swirling into your body.

- Now imagine the carbon dioxide in your exhalation as it moves back up and out of your body, taking with it any tension, discomfort, pain, or illness.

- Bring your awareness now to your abdomen. Imagine a pair of nostrils in the middle of your belly through which you are now breathing. Visualize the oxygen coming in and swirling all around your abdomen, bowel, inner organs, and lower back, bringing healing energy with it. Imagine the oxygen and life force penetrating deep into areas of darkness or stagnation, refreshing you and healing you. As you exhale through the imaginary nostrils in your belly, visualize any tension, pain, or negative feelings flowing up and out of your body to be released.

- Now visualize a pair of nostrils in the center of your chest, near your heart, through which you are now breathing. Imagine the oxygen and life force swirling all around your chest, your ribs, your shoulders, and your back, delivering oxygen and healing energy. As you exhale through the imaginary nostrils near your heart, imagine all the stress, negative emotions, and anxiety leaving your body.

- Now, bring your awareness to a part of your body that is tense, tired, or in some discomfort or pain. Visualize a pair of nostrils located right in the middle of this point. Imagine the oxygen and life force entering the nostrils and swirling all around the area of tension, pain, or discomfort. With each inhalation, healing energy is swirling in and permeating every cell in that area. With each exhalation, tension, pain or impurities are taken away, leaving that part of your body refreshed, cleansed, and healed.

- Continue this visualization technique, breathing directly into each point of discomfort in your body, delivering oxygen and healing energy, and removing all stress and anxiety.

- Bring your awareness now to the center of your forehead. Visualize the air entering your body here through imaginary nostrils. See the oxygen and lifeforce-rich air swirling around, dissolving any tension behind the eyes and in all the muscles of your face. As you exhale, imagine all the stress and tension being carried away and released.

- Now, bring your attention to the crown of your head—where a small pair of nostrils is breathing in nutrient-rich oxygen and *prana*. Visualize this breath as a soft white mist, swirling down through the top of your head and spreading across your face, neck, shoulders, arms, chest, back, buttocks, thighs, knees, calves, feet, and right down to your toes. Continue to breathe in and out until this white mist fills your body from head to toe. As you breathe in and out, let this white mist flow all the way down your spine and out again. Visualize this mist swirling around your body, removing all remaining stress or tension. Allow yourself to experience the calmness and vitality this exercise can bring you.

- Then, when you are ready, begin to breathe normally. Give your body a stretch and slowly open your eyes. Allow yourself a few moments to reorient yourself before getting up. Be aware that this feeling of well-being will remain with you for the rest of the day.

PART THREE

THE FIVE
TIBETAN RITES

THE EYE OF REVELATION
1939 & 1946 EDITIONS COMBINED
The True Five Tibetan Rites

AUTHOR'S NOTE

The following pages include extracts from my book, *The Eye of Revelation 1939 & 1946 Editions Combined.* It is the only book that compares both versions of the original book by Peter Kelder, published in 1939 and updated in 1946. These two editions are significant as they represent the evolution and refinement of the Five Tibetan Exercises over time.

Since this book is about enhancing the Five Tibetan Exercises with breathing techniques, I have only included extracts and information from the original text that relate to the context of this book. I have also included practical tips and information from my twenty-three years of teaching practice. These insights have been gleaned from thousands of students' experiences in learning and practicing the Rites and I'm sure they will help you with your practice.

INTRODUCTION

*T*he *Eye of Revelation* is a compelling and long-lasting account of a Westerner known only as 'Colonel Bradford,' who discovered a secret sect of monks living in a remote Tibetan monastery. Despite their advanced years, these monks were remarkably healthy and youthful. Bradford lived and studied with the monks for several years, where they taught him their secret to what some refer to as the 'fountain of youth.' Bradford brought this knowledge back to the West, where it became known as 'The Five Tibetan Rites of Rejuvenation.'

As a long-term teacher of the Rites over the last twenty-three years, I have always found it essential to know Kelder's true words. I found it fascinating to compare his original 1939 and 1946 updated editions in great detail and see what he added and removed from the original text. For example, Kelder never used the word 'chakras' when referring to what he described as magnetic centers. He called them 'vortexes.'

This book contains Kelder's words and illustrations precisely as he created them long ago - reproduced here from the scans of rare books - the 1939 & 1946 editions of The Eye of Revelation, owned by the late antiquarian book collector and seller Jerry Watt (RIP). Jerry and I shared a desire to keep the original words intact, and he gave me his scans with full permission to publish them as I saw fit.

I hope you will find some of the tips I have shared with you useful and interesting. These include practice tips, additional information, and suggestions on what to avoid when learning the Rites. There isn't space in this book to teach you all I know about learning and practicing the Five Tibetan Rites, so if you need more in-depth information, my book, *The Illustrated Five Tibetan Rites*, or my online training course may be helpful to learn from.

NOTE:

- Any important changes Kelder added or deleted in his updated 1946 Edition are highlighted in bold or included in square brackets.
- Some of these are significant changes and will provide insights into what Kelder considered essential and what he felt needed changing.
- Most of Kelder's changes to his 1946 update were additional instructions on how to perform the Rites. The publisher's foreword below was also significantly changed.
- I have <u>not changed</u> Kelder's text at all, and some of you will notice punctuation and grammatical errors, which I have not corrected. This is intentional, as I believe it adds a greater sense of time and place to the story.
- I have used *italics* to distinguish my added content from the original.

FOREWORD BY THE ORIGINAL PUBLISHERS 1939 EDITION

Note: *The text in bold below was deleted from the 1946 update. The most significant alteration is the change of wording from* **25 centuries to just 'centuries'** *for the date of origin of the Rites.*

"*THE EYE OF REVELATION*" is truly a revelation. It reveals **to you** information which has been known and used by men in far-distant lands for **more than 25** centuries, **but which is now available to you for the first time.** Information which has been thoroughly tried and tested **and which has been proven beyond a doubt to be the greatest gift ever bestowed on man in this material plane of existence.** Information that will stem the tide of premature old age with its attendant weaknesses and senility.

This is the information for which Ponce de Leon, and thousands of others down through the ages, would have given all they possessed; **for with such information they quickly could have regained all that they had paid and more.**

"*THE EYE OF REVELATION*" [**"will often"** was added to the 1946 Edition] produces remarkable mental and physical rejuvenation within a month. So much so, in fact, that one gains new hope and enthusiasm, with which to carry on.

However, the greatest results come after the tenth week. When you stop to consider that the average man ["man" was replaced with **person** in the 1946 Edition] has endured his afflictions from 20 to 30 years, to obtain such amazing results in such a short time as **ten** weeks sounds almost miraculous.

There is positively no limit to the improvement and progress one can make with this information. As long as you live and practice *"THE EYE OF REVELATION"* you will get more gratifying results. **Not only will they be manifested in the material, but if the fortunate individual so desires he may improve his mental world as well as all the other worlds to which man is heir.**

MOST IMPORTANT: The information given in *"THE EYE OF REVELATION"* was, for **twenty-five centuries**, confined strictly to men. Now, to the surprise and delight of all concerned, it has been found that women, too, get equally beneficial and amazing results. **Now, after this long period of waiting every adult, man or woman,** can go on to grand and glorious things, regardless of **age**, environment or circumstances.

Get started at once on the marvellous work of REJUVE-NATION, TRANSMUTATION and *YOUTHIFICATION*, May success, health, energy, power, vigor, virility, and *LIFE* follow your footsteps forever.

THE PUBLISHERS

10

COLONEL BRADFORD'S GREAT DISCOVERY

One afternoon I dropped into the Travelers Club to escape a sudden shower, and while seated in an easy chair I fell into conversation with a most interesting old gentleman; one who, although I did not know it then, was destined to change the whole course of my life. I call him an old man for that is exactly what he was. In his late sixties, he looked every year his age. He was thin and stooped, and when he walked leaned heavily on his cane.

It developed that he was a retired British army officer, who had likewise seen service in the diplomatic corps of the Crown. There were few accessible places on the globe to which Colonel Bradford, as I shall call him, although that was not his true name, had not, at some time or other in his life, paid a visit, and warming under my attention, he related incidents in his travels which were highly entertaining. Needless to say, I spent an interesting and profitable afternoon, listening to him. This was some years ago. We met often after that and got along famously. Many evenings, either at his quarters or at mine, we discussed and discoursed until long past midnight.

It was on one of these occasions I became possessed of a feeling that Colonel Bradford wanted to tell me something of importance. Something close to his heart which was difficult for him to talk about. By using all the tact and diplomacy at my command I succeeded in making him understand that I should be happy to help him in any way possible, and that if he cared to tell me what was on his mind I would keep it in strict confidence. Slowly at first, and then with increased trust he began to talk.

While stationed in India some years ago, Colonel Bradford, from time to time, came in contact with wandering natives from the remote fastnesses of the country. He heard many interesting tales of the life and customs of the country. One story, which interested him strangely, he heard quite a number of times, and always from natives who inhabited a particular district. Those from other districts never seemed to have heard this story.

It concerned a group of Lamas or Tibetan priests who, apparently, had discovered "The Fountain of Youth." The natives told of old men who had mysteriously regained health and vigor, strength and virility shortly after entering a certain Lamasery; but where this particular place was none seemed exactly to know.

Like so many other men, Colonel Bradford had become old at 40, and had not been getting any younger as the years rolled by. Now the more he heard this tale of "The Fountain of Youth" the more he became convinced that such a place and such men actually existed. He began to gather information on directions, character of the country, climate, and various other tid-bits that might help him locate the spot; for from then on there dwelt in the back of his mind a desire to find this "Fountain of Youth."

This desire, he told me, had now grown so powerful that he had determined to return to India and start in earnest a quest for the retreat of the young-old men; and he wanted me to go with him. Frankly, by the time he had finished telling me this fantastic story I, too, was convinced of its truth, and was half-tempted to join him, but I finally decided against it.

Soon he departed, and I consoled myself for not going with the thought that perhaps one should be satisfied to grow old gracefully; that perhaps the Colonel was wrong in trying to get more out of life than was vouchsafed to other men. And yet – a Fountain of Youth!!! What a thrilling idea it was! For his own sake I hoped that the old Colonel might find it.

Months passed. In the press of every-day affairs Colonel Bradford and his "Shangri-La" had grown dim in my memory, when one evening on returning to my apartment, there was a letter in the Colonel's own handwriting. He was still alive! The letter seemed to have been written in joyous desperation. In it he said that in spite of maddening delays and set-backs he actually was on the verge of finding the "Fountain." He gave no address.

It was more months before I heard from him again. This time he had good news. He had found the "Fountain of Youth"! Not only that, but he was bringing it back to the States with him, and would arrive within the next two months. Practically four years had elapsed since I had last seen the old man. Would he have changed any, I wondered? He was older, of course, but perhaps no balder, although his stoop might have increased a little. Then the startling idea came to me that perhaps this "Fountain of Youth" might really have helped him. But in my mind's eye I could not picture him differently than I had seen him last, except perhaps a little older.

One evening I decided to stay at home by myself and catch up on my reading, maybe write a few letters. I had finally settled down to comfortable reading when the telephone rang.

"A Colonel Bradford to see you, sir," said the desk clerk.

"Send him up," I shouted, and casting the book aside I hastened to the door. In a short time a rap was heard on the door. I opened it in haste. For a moment I stared, and then with dismay I saw that this was not Colonel Bradford, but a much younger man.

Noting my surprise he said, "Weren't you expecting me?"

"No," I confessed. "I thought it would be an old friend of mine, a Colonel Bradford."

"I came to see you about Colonel Bradford, the man you were expecting," he answered.

"Come in," I invited.

"Allow me to introduce myself," said the stranger, entering. "My name is Bradford."

"Oh, you are Colonel Bradford's son," I exclaimed. "I have often heard him speak of you so often. You resemble him somewhat."

"No, I am not my son," he returned. "I am none other than your old friend, Colonel Bradford, the old man who went away to the Himalayas."

I stood in incredulous amazement at his statement. Then it slowly dawned upon me that this really was the Colonel Bradford whom I had known; but what a change had taken place in his appearance. Instead of the stooped, limping, sallow old gentleman with a cane, he was a tall, straight, ruddy-complexioned man in the prime of life.[1] Even his hair, which had grown back, held only a trace of grey.[2]

(1)   *The Rites improve your posture by strengthening your back and abdominal muscles so you can hold yourself erect. Together with a conscious decision to remove "old people mannerisms" from yourself, like stooping, slumping, dithering, etc., you'll feel more energetic, and people will say how much younger you look. You'll feel it too.*

(2) *I don't want to disillusion anyone, but I have only once seen a mild change in hair color. The sideburns of one of my students appeared to have darkened after several months of practice. Going from completely grey to completely dark is probably unrealistic, and if it happened regularly would be reported on the front-page news!*

My enthusiasm and curiosity knew no bounds. Soon I was plying him with questions in rapid-fire order until he threw up his hands.

"Wait, wait," he protested, laughingly. "I shall start at the beginning and tell you all that has happened." And this he proceeded to do.

Upon arriving in India the Colonel started directly for the district in which lived the natives who had told of "The Fountain of Youth." Fortunately, he knew quite a bit of their language. He spent a number of months there, making friends with the people and picking up all the information he could about the Lamasery he sought. It was a long, slow process, but his shrewdness and persistence finally brought him to the coveted place he had heard about so often, but only half-believed existed.

Colonel Bradford's account of what transpired after being admitted to the Lamasery sounded like a fairy tale. I only wish that time and space permitted me to set down here all of his experiences; the interesting practices of the Lamas, their culture, and their utter indifference to the work-a-day world. There were no real old men there. To his surprise the Lamas considered Colonel Bradford a quite novel sight, for it had been a long time since they had seen anyone who looked as old as he. The Lamas good-naturedly referred to the Colonel as "The Ancient One."

"For the first two weeks after I arrived," said the Colonel, "I was like a fish out of water. I marvelled at everything I saw, and at times could hardly believe what my eyes beheld. I soon felt much better, was sleeping like a top every night, and only used my cane when hiking in the mountains.

"A month after I arrived I received the biggest surprise of my life. In fact, I was quite startled. It was the day I entered for the first time, a large, well-ordered room which was used as a kind of library for ancient manuscripts. At one end of the room was a full-length mirror. It had been over two years since I had last seen my reflection, so with great curiosity I stepped in front of the glass.

"I stared in amazement, so changed was my appearance. It seemed that I had dropped 15 years from my age. It was my first intimation that I was growing younger; but from then on I changed so rapidly that it was apparent to all who knew me. Soon the honorary title of "The Ancient One" was heard no more."

A knock at the door interrupted the Colonel. I opened it to admit a couple of friends from out of town who had picked this most inauspicious time to spend a sociable evening with me. I hid my disappointment and chagrin as best I could and introduced them to Colonel Bradford. We all chatted together for a while, and then the Colonel said, rising:

"I am sorry that I must leave so early, but I have an appointment with an old friend who is leaving the city tonight. I hope I shall see you all again shortly."

At the door he turned to me and said, softly, "Could you have lunch with me tomorrow? I promise, if you can do so, you shall hear all about "The Fountain of Youth.""

We agreed as to the time and place and the Colonel departed. As I returned to the living room, one of my friends remarked,

"That is certainly a most interesting man, but he looks awfully young to be retired from army service."

"How old do you suppose he is?" I asked.

"Well, he doesn't look forty," answered my friend, "but from the experiences he has had I suppose he must be that old."

"Yes, he's all of that," I replied evasively, and deftly turned the conversation into another channel. I thought it best to arouse no wonderment regarding the Colonel until I knew what his plans were.

The next day, after having lunch together, we repaired to the Colonel's room in a nearby hotel, and there at last he told me about "The Fountain of Youth."

"The first important thing I was taught after entering the Lamasery," he began, "was this. The body has seven centers, which, in English, could be called Vortexes. These are kind of magnetic centers. They revolve at great speed in the healthy body, but when slowed down – well, that is just another name for old age, ill-health, and senility. "There are two of these Vortexes in the brain; one at the base of the throat; another in the right side of the body in the region of the liver; one in the sexual center; and one in each knee.

"These spinning centers of activity extend beyond the flesh in the healthy individual, but in the old, weak, senile person they hardly reach the surface, except in the knees. The quickest way to regain health, youth, and vitality is to start these magnetic centers spinning again. "There are but five practices that will do this. Any one of them ["especially the first" – added to the 1946 Edition] will be helpful, but all five are required to get glowing results. These five exercises are really not exercises at all, in the physical culture sense. The Lamas think of them as 'Rites,' and so instead of calling them exercises or practices, we too, shall call them Rites."

THERE ARE SEVEN PSYCHIC VORTEXES IN THE PHYSICAL BODY

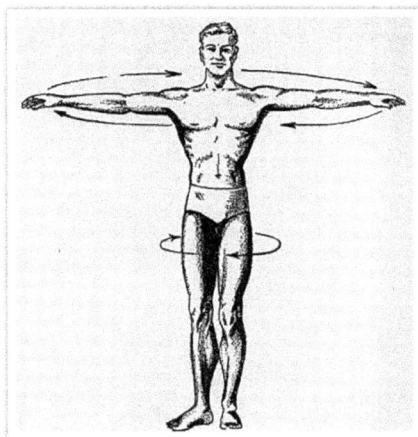

There are SEVEN Psychic Vortexes in the physical body. Vortex "A" is located within the forehead; Vortex "B" is located in the posterior part of the brain; Vortex "C" is in the region of the throat at the base of the neck; Vortex "D" is located in the right side of the body above the waist line; Vortex "E" is located in the reproductive anatomy, **and it is directly connected with Vortex "C" in the throat.** Vortexes "F" and "G" are located in either knee.

These Psychic Vortexes revolve at great speed. When all are revolving at the same speed the body is in good health. When one or more of them slow down, old age, loss of power, or senility begin to set in ("almost immediately" – added to 1946 Edition.)

- **Vortex "A"** is located deep within the forehead.
- **Vortex "B"** is in the posterior part of the brain.

- **Vortex "C"** located in the throat at the base of the neck.
- **Vortex "D"** located in the right side of the body (waist line).
- **Vortex "E"** is in the reproductive anatomy or organs.
- **Vortexes "F"** and **"G"** located one in either knee.

The list of Vortexes above was added to the 1946 Edition

11

THE BENEFITS OF THE FIVE TIBETAN RITES

The reasons why people learn and practice the Rites, is because they –

Are attracted to the anti-aging benefits of the Rites.

Have noticed the first signs of aging and want to do whatever they can to stop-the-clock.

Wish to increase their energy, mental agility and focus.

Want a simple, daily routine that improves motivation, mood and purpose.

Want to maintain a regular exercise routine, and adopt a healthier lifestyle.

Want to improve their strength and flexibility.

Lead busy lives, and want a form of exercise that fits into their daily routine. They like the fact that the Five Rites take just 10 to 15 minutes per day to practice once learned.

Want to strengthen their backs to reduce back-ache or rehabilitate an injury (with doctor's approval.)

Like the idea of practicing yoga, but don't have the time or perhaps desire to attend classes.

Like the fact the Five Rites can be done anywhere, at any time. No special equipment or facilities needed.

The typical benefits people receive from doing the Rites vary from person to person. For some, the effects are dramatic, and for others, the improvements they notice at the beginning soon become part of their normal physiology. Others may not experience much of a change at all but describe a strong sense that the Rites are improving their health and vitality.

The cumulative benefits, however, do seem to continue, and there are many people in their 70s to 90s still doing the Rites after 20 or 30 years of practice.

Mention must be made here of exaggerated claims about the benefits of the Rites that have proliferated over the internet. This appears to have started when online marketers began selling a version of "The Eye of Revelation" on a commission basis. They had no experience in teaching the Rites and may not have practiced them personally. Some certainly didn't, promoting the Rites as some kind of miracle cure.

People were led to believe that the Rites would completely halt their aging, help them lose enormous amounts of weight, and fix their cancer, heart disease, fibroid cysts, and numerous other serious health conditions. This diluted the Rites' credibility and increased people's expectations so high that disillusionment was inevitable. Anything short of a miracle was therefore seen as somewhat ho-hum.

In fact, the monks who developed the Rites didn't describe specific benefits—they simply stated that the specific purpose of the Rites is to regain health, youth, and vitality:

> "The body has seven centers, which, in English, could be called Vortexes. These are kind of magnetic centers. They revolve at great speed in the healthy body, but when slowed down – well, that is just another name for old age, ill-health, and senility. The quickest way to regain health, youth, and vitality is to start these magnetic centers

spinning again. There are but five practices that will do this. Any one of them will be helpful, but all five are required to get glowing results. These five exercises are really not exercises at all, in the physical culture sense. The Lamas think of them as 'Rites,' and so instead of calling them exercises or practices, we too shall call them 'Rites.'"

—**Peter Kelder**, *The Eye of Revelation.*

THE POWER OF BELIEF

While it is important to have realistic expectations, the power of belief (or faith) is still a vital force. Colonel Bradford, the principal character of this story said you need to invest a strong amount of faith and belief in the Rites to maximize their benefit. If you think old, you behave old, for example. Standing up straight is one of the most effective ways to appear younger, and these exercises will help improve your posture to achieve that.

A good example of this is the medical use of placebos. A common practice is to give patients an inert sugar pill without telling them the pill is a placebo. Having been told the pill will improve their condition, the patient's belief does indeed have a therapeutic effect, improving the condition it was intended for.

WHAT KIND OF BENEFITS CAN YOU EXPECT?

To produce this list, I have only reported benefits that I can directly verify or confirm. I have not used any second or third–hand sources of information and have compiled the benefits on this list from the feedback forms of hundreds of students who attended our Five Tibetan Rites workshops. It includes testimonials from people who have learned the Rites from my books, DVD or Online Training Course.

A significant increase in energy – more the endurance type of energy than the revved-up caffeine type. You feel like you can keep going and going.

Feel calmer and less stressed – your buttons simply don't get pushed as easily anymore.

Develop significant mental clarity with razor-sharp focus.

Feel stronger, more flexible, and less stiff.

Enjoy seeing muscles appear on your arms, stomachs, hips, legs, and backs. Good for toning flabby arms and tightening the abdomen.

Sleep better. Some people have more vivid dreams.

Overall improvement in your health, don't seem to catch colds, etc., as often. Helps with depression and anxiety – lifts mood and improves well-being. More centered and at peace.

Improved self-discipline and sense of purpose.

Feel younger and more powerful.

Improved breathing – deeper, slower, and more conscious.

Increased levels of Qi (chi, prana, life-energy).

Better posture.

Develops good core strength, which provides a strong foundation for any other form of exercise or modern living.

Some people lose weight; most find it easier to control weight and desire healthier foods.

Improved digestion and elimination.

Helps with the transition and symptoms of menopause.

Helps with the symptoms of menstruation.

Improved libido.

Many people also claim the Rites have made significant improvements to their health conditions. You can read their testimonials **on the** *T5T website.*

HEALTH CONSIDERATIONS

W henever you begin a new exercise program, there are always health considerations to consider. The information in this section is not comprehensive, and you should not substitute it for the direct advice of your doctor or health care provider.

If you feel any unusual discomfort or pain when you begin the Rites, stop practicing the exercises immediately and discuss the situation with your qualified healthcare provider. If you have had a previous injury or are suffering from one at the moment, you must check with your health practitioner to ensure that the Rites will not aggravate your injury. Also, if you have a history of knee, shoulder, back, or neck injuries, it is always advisable to consult a qualified medical professional before attempting any of the postures.

PREGNANCY

It's important to note that the Rites are not intended for pregnant women, as this is not the best time for you to begin a new workout program, particularly without the advice of a qualified health or fitness professional. If you are pregnant and have already been practicing yoga or Pilates regularly, you should discuss this program with a qualified prenatal yoga or Pilates Instructor, as modifications or alterations may be possible. However, some of *these exercises are not recommended, particularly in late-term. Once your baby is delivered, you'll find that the exercises are an excellent way to get yourself back into shape, and they can be done while the baby sleeps – or at a time that suits you.*

COMPARISONS BETWEEN THE ORIGINAL 1939 EDITION AND THE 1946 UPDATE

I have carefully compared the original 1939 version of 'The Eye of Revelation' to Peter Kelder's 1946 update in great detail. Other than minor word replacements, Kelder's most significant changes were to his instructions on performing Rites Nos 1-5. In the initial 1939 version, there were no instructions beneath the images for each Rite, whereas in the 1946 version, Kelder has added new information. I have highlighted these changes in bold so you can compare them.

1. **1939 Edition:** Kelder provides one or two illustrations and a story about each Rite. His descriptions are very brief, with just a few lines describing how to perform each movement.

2. **1946 Edition:** Beneath the same images as in the 1939 version, Kelder added additional instructions and some amendments.

3. I have used **bold or square brackets** to highlight these changes so you know what Kelder considered important enough to change.

4. I have not highlighted the few minor word changes he made, such as replacing the word "direction" with the word "way."

14

THE FIVE TIBETAN RITES Nos 1-5

BUILDING REPETITIONS

"To start with," said he, "I would suggest you practice each Rite three times a day for the first week. Then increase them by two a day each week until you are doing 21 a day, which will be at the beginning of the 10th week."

—**Colonel Bradford** in *The Eye of Revelation.*

I recommend you follow Bradford's instructions to build up repetitions as he describes above. Many changes occur in the body, and it takes time to adjust. You can feel unbalanced, not present, scattered, or moody when you do too many repetitions too quickly.

Some people are very keen to reach 21 repetitions as quickly as possible, but I can assure you that most of the gifts happen during the journey. Remember to enjoy the journey – your achievement will be more rewarding if you do so.

ADDING ENERGY BREATHING

There are three steps to Energy Breathing as you have already learned. For the first three weeks of your practice you move through Steps 1-3 and then remain on Step 3 indefinitely.

Week	Repetitions of Each Rite	Energy Breathing Steps
1	3 x	1
2	5 x	2
3	7 x	3
4	9 x	3
5	11 x	3
6	13 x	3
7	15 x	3
8	17 x	3
9	19 x	3
10	21 x	3

THE FIVE TIBETAN RITES ON ONE PAGE

*Most people find it helpful to have the full sequence from Rites 1-5 on one page – see images below. You can **also download and print** these posters for free on the T5T.com website (T5T is short for The Five Tibetans.)*

T5T The Five Tibetan Rites

www.T5T.com

Courses, books, DVD, Videos, Free Resources

1 The Spin — Energy — I am full of energy

2 Leg Raise — Air — My mind is clear and calm

3 Kneeling Backbend — Water — I am flexible and receptive

4 Table Top — Earth — I am strong and balanced

5 Pendulum — Fire — I am positive and motivated

© Carolinda Witt 2023

RITE
NUMBER ONE

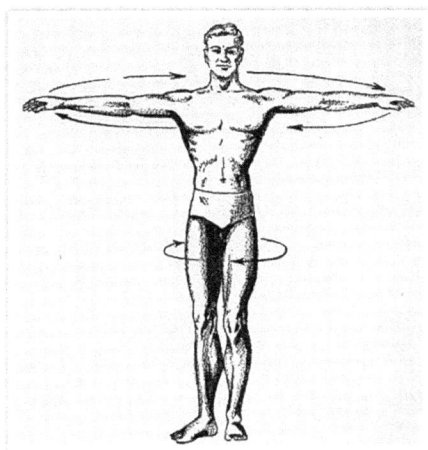

" The first Rite," continued the Colonel "is a simple one. It is for the express purpose of speeding up the Vortexes. When we were children we used it in our play. It is this:

"Stand erect with arms outstretched, horizontal with the shoulders. Now spin around until you become slightly dizzy. There is only one caution: you must turn from left to right. In other words, if you were to place a clock or watch on the floor face up, you would turn in the same direction the hands are moving." *(1939 & 1946 Editions – Introduction.)*

> **Energy Breathing**
>
> - *When you stop, immediately stand with your legs hip-width apart, knees slightly bent, and your hands on your hips. Allow any dizziness to dissipate, then wrap your hands around your ribs in the Energy Breathing position.*
>
> - *Breathe out, then complete three Energy Breaths,* **Steps 1, 2,** *or* **3,** *ending with an inhalation (see Chapter 8). Wait until all dizziness disappears before beginning Rite No. 2 - The Leg Raise.*

"At first the average adult will only be able to "spin around" about a half-dozen times until he becomes dizzy enough to want to sit or lie down. That is just what he should do, too. That's what I did. To begin with, practice this Rite only to the point of slight dizziness.[3] As time passes and your Vortexes become more rapid in movement through this and other Rites, you will be able to practice it to a greater extent.

"When I was in India it amazed me to see the *Maulawiyah*, or as they are more commonly known, the Whirling Dervishes, almost unceasingly spin around and around in a religious frenzy.

(Mawlawīyah, Turkish Mevleviyah, a fraternity of Sufis (Muslim mystics) founded in Konya (Qonya), Anatolia, by the Persian Sufi poet Rūmī (d. 1273), whose popular title mawlānā (Arabic: "our master") gave the order its name.) – **Encyclopedia Britannica**

"Rite Number One recalled to my attention two things in connection with this practice. The first was that these Whirling Dervishes always spun in one direction – from left to right, or clockwise.

In fact, the Dervishes **spin counterclockwise**, *not clockwise, as described by Kelder above. Rumi's family describe the spin direction of the Dervishes during the "Sema," a religious ceremony carried out in remembrance of God below.*

"Revolving around the heart, from right to left, he embraces all the mankind, all the creation with affection and love."

—**Rumi's family** – Mevlana.net

"The second was the virility of the old men; they were strong, hearty, and robust. Far more than most Englishmen are at their age.

"When I spoke to one of the Lamas about this, he informed me that while this whirling movement of the Dervishes did have a very beneficial effect, yet it also had a devastating one. It seems that a long siege of whirling stimulates into great activity Vortexes "A," "B," and "E." These three have a stimulating effect on the other two – "C" and "D." But due to excessive leg action the Vortexes in the knees – "E" and "G" – are over-stimulated and finally so exhausted that the building up of the Vital Forces along with this tearing down causes the participants to experience a kind of "psychic jag" which they mistake for something very spiritual ["or at least religious" – added to the 1946 Edition.]

"However," continued the Colonel, "we do not carry the whirling exercise to excess. While the whirling Dervishes may spin around many hundreds of times, we find that greater benefit is obtained by restricting it to about a dozen or so times, or enough so that Rite Number One can stimulate all the Vortexes to action." ["After several months it can be increased to 20 revolutions. Later to 30, 40, and eventually, after many months, to 50" – added to the 1946 Edition.]

(3) *If you experience dizziness, don't be disheartened as it usually improves over time. I have seen fit people, and those who practice yoga regularly (including teachers) take around six months to build up to 21 repetitions of the spin because of dizziness. By far, the vast majority of people have no trouble at all unless they try to do too many repetitions too quickly.*

The symptoms of dizziness/motion sickness occur because your brain receives conflicting information from your sensory systems. These senses send information to your brain about the position and movement of your body. This includes your eyes, the sensors of the semicircular canals in your inner ears, and the somatosensory receptors in your skin, joints, and muscles. A mismatch in sensory information causes a conflict between what is seen or felt and your previous orientational experience. When this happens, the body responds with the symptoms of dizziness and motion sickness. For this reason, using the correct technique during the spin is crucial.

To reduce dizziness, try fine-tuning your movements by using the techniques described in **Appendix (A)**, *at the back of this book.*

ALTERNATIVE TO THE SPIN

In the rare likelihood that dizziness becomes a problem for you – try this alternative.

Simply swing your arms at shoulder height around to the opposite shoulder, and repeat to the other side. Your head and upper body twist around to one side and then the other. Your feet remain stationary, but remember to lift the opposite heel to the direction you are turning to avoid straining your lower back.

There is no twisting movement in The Five Tibetan Rites, so this exercise improves flexibility and reduces tension. I do it every day because it feels so good.

RITE
NUMBER TWO

"Like Rite Number One," continued the Colonel, "this second one is for further stimulating to action the Seven Vortexes. It is even simpler than the first one. In Rite Number Two one first lies flat on his back on the floor or on the bed.[4] If practiced on the floor one should use a rug or blanket under him, folded several times in order that the body will not come into contact with the cold floor. The Lamas have what in English might be called a 'prayer rug.' It is about two feet wide and fully six feet long. It is fairly thick and is made from wool and a kind of vegetable fibre. It is solely for the purpose of insulation, and so has no other value. Nevertheless, to the Lamas everything is of a religious nature, hence their name for these mats – 'prayer rugs.'

"As I said, one should lie full length on his 'prayer rug' or bed. Then place the hands flat down alongside the hips. The fingers should be kept close together with the fingertips of each hand turned slightly toward one another. The feet are then raised until the legs are straight up. If possible, let the feet extend back a bit over the body, toward the head; but do not let the knees bend. Then, slowly lower the feet to the floor and for a moment allow all muscles to relax. Then perform this Rite all over again.

"One of the Lamas told me that when he first attempted to practice this simple Rite he was so old, weak, and decrepit that he couldn't possibly lift up both legs. Therefore he started out by lifting the thighs until the knees were straight up, letting the feet hang down. Little by little, however, he was able to straighten out his legs until eventually he could raise them straight with perfect ease.

"I marveled at this particular Lama," said the Colonel, "when he told me this. He was then a perfect picture of health and youth, although I knew he was many years older than I. For the sheer joy of exerting himself, he used to carry up a pack of vegetables weighing fully a hundred pounds on his back, from the garden to the Lamasery, several hundred feet above. He took his time but never stopped once on the way up, and when he would arrive he didn't seem to be experiencing the slightest bit of fatigue. I marveled greatly at this, for the first time I started up with him, and I was carrying no load, I had to stop at least a dozen times. Later I was able to do it easily without my cane and with never a stop, but that is another story."

(4) *Avoid practicing the Leg Raise on your bed unless your bed is very firm. Any sagging in the mattress caused by your body weight changes your spine's natural and optimal S-shape, creating additional strain on the supporting muscles that protect your pelvis, neck, and spine. Since these movements are done repetitively, you should do Rite No 2 on the floor, using a yoga mat, rug, or carpet for comfort.*

RITE NO 2 – THE LEG RAISE

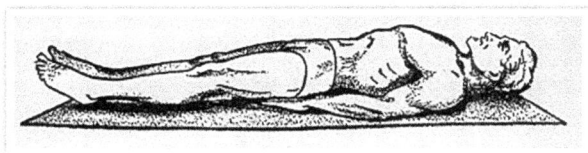

First Position of Rite No. 2

"One should lie full length on his 'prayer-rug,' or bed. Then place the hands flat alongside the hips. Fingers should be kept close together with the finger-tips of each hand turned slightly toward one another." (*1939 & 1946 Editions – Introduction.*)

"To perform this Rite lie full length on rug or bed. Place the hands **flat down** alongside of the hips. Fingers should be kept close together with the finger-tips of each hand turned slightly toward one another." (*1946 Edition – New information is in bold.*)

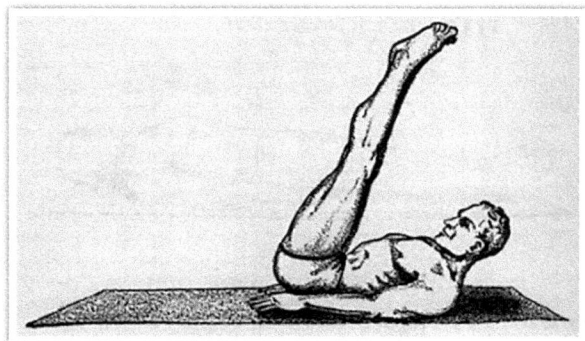

Second Position of Rite No. 2

"The feet are then raised until the legs are straight up. If possible, let the feet extend back a bit over the body, toward the head; but do not let the knees bend. Then, slowly lower the feet to the floor and for a moment allow all muscles to relax. Then perform this Rite all over again." (*1939 & 1946 Editions – Introduction.*)

"Raise the feet until the legs are straight up. If possible, let the feet extend back a bit over the body toward the head, but do not let the knees bend.[5] **Hold this position for a moment or two** and then slowly lower the feet to the floor, and for the **next several** moments allow all of the muscles **in the entire body to relax completely**. Then perform this Rite all over again.

While the feet and legs are being raised it is a good idea also to raise the head, then while the feet and legs are being lowered to the floor lower the head at the same time.

By raising the head at the same time the legs and feet are raised all of the Vortexes in the body are increased in their speed or action, but especially the slow ones." (*1946 Edition – New information is in bold.*)

Energy Breathing

- *Remain lying on your back, bend your knees and place your hands in the Energy Breathing Position with your hands wrapped around your lower ribs.*
- *Exhale fully, then take three complete Energy Breaths, **Steps 1, 2,** or **3**, ending with an inhalation (see Chapter 8).*

(5)   *If you have suffered back pain in the past or are unfit, I recommend you avoid bringing your legs back over the stomach, as illustrated above, as it takes the spine out of its natural 'neutral' position. Neutral spine is a term used to describe the natural S-shape of the spine when its natural curves are maintained. The muscles closest to the spine (the core muscles) are more effective at stabilizing and protecting the spine (like guide wires on a tent) when the spine is in neutral.*

When you bring your legs back over your stomach, as illustrated above, your tailbone lifts and the curve of your lower back is flattened to the floor. Instead, only raise your legs to a point where your knee bones are aligned over your hip bones (joint over joint), and the natural curve of your lower back remains intact. It makes no difference to the benefits of the Rites if you don't bring your legs back over your stomach.

If you need to bend your knees initially and then gradually straighten them as your flexibility increases, this is preferable to straining your lower back or neck.

RITE
NUMBER THREE

" The third Rite should be practiced immediately after practicing Rite Number Two. It, too, is a very simple one. All one needs to do is to kneel on his 'prayer rug,' place his hands on his thighs, and lean forward as far as possible with the head inclined so that the chin rests on the chest. Now lean backward as far as possible; at the same time the head should be lifted and thrown back as far as it will go. Then bring the head up along with the body. Lean forward again and start the rite all over. This Rite is very effective in speeding up Vortexes 'E,' 'D,' and 'C'; especially 'E.'

"I have seen more than 200 Lamas perform this Rite together. In order to turn their attention within, they closed their eyes. In this way they would not become confused by what others were doing and thus have their attention diverted.

"The Lamas, millenniums ago, discovered that all good things come from within. They discovered that every worthwhile thing has its origin within the individual. This is something that the Occidental has never been able to understand and comprehend. He thinks, as I did, that all worthwhile things must come from the outside world.

"The Lamas, especially those at this particular Lamasery, are performing a great work for the world. It is performed, however, on the astral plane. This plane, from which they assist mankind in all quarters of the globe, is high enough above the vibrations of the world to be a powerful focal point where much can be accomplished with little loss of effort.

"Someday the world will awaken in amazement to what the unseen forces – the Forces of Good – have been doing for the masses. We who take ourselves in hand and make new creatures of ourselves in every imaginable way, each is doing a marvelous work for mankind everywhere. Already the efforts of these advanced individuals are being welded together into One Irresistible Power. A new day is dawning for the world – it is already here. But it is only through individuals like the Lamas, and you and me, that the world can possibly be helped.

"Most of mankind, and that includes those in the most enlightened countries, like America, Canada and England, is still in the darkest of the Dark Ages. However, they are being prepared for better and more glorious things, and as fast as they can be initiated into the higher life, just that fast will the world be made a better place in which to live."

RITE NO 3 – THE KNEELING BACKBEND

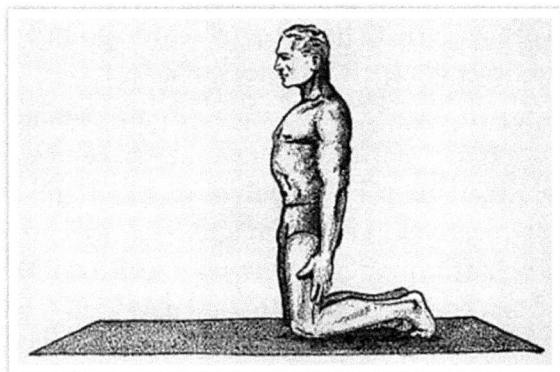

First Position of Rite No. 3

"The third Rite should be practiced immediately after one practices Rite Number Two. It, too, is a very simple one. All one needs to do is kneel on his 'prayer rug,' place his hands on his thighs, and lean forward as far as possible with the head inclined so that the chin rests on the chest." (*1939 & 1946 Editions – Introduction.*)

"The first position of this Rite is to kneel on a rug or mat **with hands at sides, palms flat against the side of the legs**. Then lean forward as far as possible,[6] **bending at the waist, with head well forward – chin on chest**." (*1946 Edition – New information is in bold.*)

(6)   *Check out the differences between the 1939 and 1946 descriptions highlighted in bold above. You will see that the illustration for the first part of Rite No 3 does not depict any*

bending at the waist, as described by Kelder. This causes confusion, so what should you do?

I recommend you learn and practice Rite No 3 without the forward bending action until your strength and flexibility increase. Once you have done so, you can experiment with the forward-bending, which doesn't appear to have any additional benefits over and above what you already receive from this Rite – at least not one you can detect.

Ideally, anyone doing this Rite should keep their spine 'long and strong' and to avoid collapsing in the lower back or neck during the movement, regardless of whether they do the forward bending movement or not. Repeatedly overbending in the lower back and neck compresses the vertebrae and discs, which can lead to strain and injury in vulnerable people – notably, older, unfit, or overweight people and anyone who has previously suffered back or neck pain.

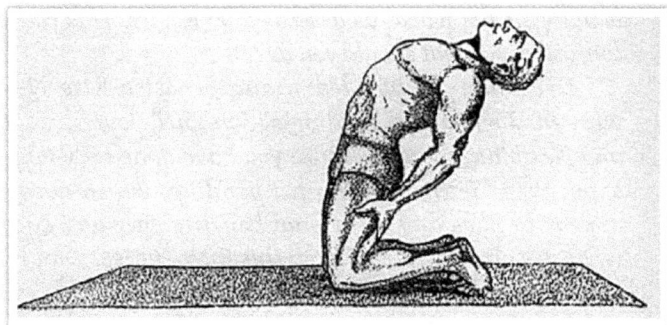

Second Position of Rite No. 3

"Now lean backward as far as possible; at the same time the head should be lifted and thrown back as far as it will go.[7] Then bring the head up along with the body. Lean forward again and start the rite all over. This Rite is very effective in speeding up Vortexes, 'E,' 'D,' and 'C'; especially 'E.'" (*1939 & 1946 Editions – Introduction.*)

"The second position of this Rite is to lean backward as far as possible.[8] **Cause the head to move still further backward. The toes will prevent you from falling over backward.**

The hands are always kept against the side of the legs. Next come to an erect (kneeling) position, relax as much as possible for a moment, and perform Rite all over again." (*1946 Edition – New information is in bold.*)

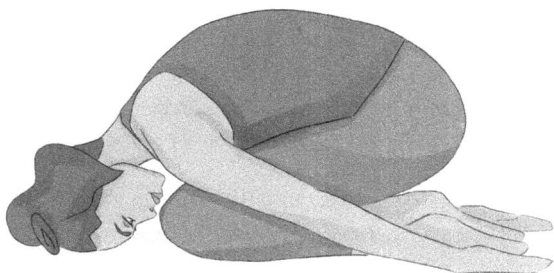

Energy Breathing

After completing the Kneeling Backbend, sit back on your heels and fold yourself forward into "Child's Pose," as illustrated above. If you can't place your forehead on the floor, make a fist (or put one fist on top of the other) and rest your head on your hand.

- *Allow your lower back to relax and stretch to compensate for the backbend you have just completed. Move your knees slightly apart to prepare for Energy Breathing. As you breathe, focus on the muscles of your back expanding and contracting with the movement of the breath.*

- *Begin by exhaling fully, then take three complete Energy Breaths, **Steps 1, 2**, or **3**, ending with an inhalation (see Chapter 8).*

- ***To get up**, place your hands on either side of your head and take a small breath, then use your hands to push yourself into an upright position, looking forward as you do so. Holding your breath until you come upright will reduce the possibility of you going red in the face or feeling a bit dizzy.*

(7)   *If you feel dizzy or faint during this movement, avoid dropping your head back "as far as it will go," as this compresses the vertebrae and discs in your neck and may occlude (kink) the vertebral artery, temporarily reducing oxygen supply to your brain. Instead, keep your neck long and strong, and don't let your head drop back so far.*

(8)   *As you can imagine, "leaning as far back as possible" creates a significant load on the lower back muscles to perform the movement and counter the effects of gravity at the same time.*

Some people lean back on their thighs to give the appearance of a deeper arch, but with repetition, the thigh and groin muscles can become strained.

Instead, keep your hip bones aligned over your knee bones and your breastbone lengthened upwards (without puffing out your ribs), as you return to the starting position. Don't collapse; maintain the length of your spine as you return to the forward starting position.

Initially, you may feel this way of doing Rite 3 is less strenuous, but this is deceptive. Try squeezing your shoulder blades together at the back as you arch backward to increase the stretch. In our daily forward-facing actions, the muscles in our shoulders and chest become stiff as very few natural movements cause us to lean backward. Take advantage of the backbend to stretch and loosen these muscles to relieve tension and increase mobility. It feels good, too.

RITE
NUMBER FOUR

"Now for Rite Number Four," said the Colonel. "The first time I tried this it seemed very difficult, but after a while it was as simple to do as any of the others.[9]

"Sit on the 'prayer rug' with the feet stretched out in front. Then place the hands alongside the body. Now raise the body and bend the knees so that the legs, from the knees down, are practically straight up and down. The arms, too, will be straight up and down, while the body, from the shoulders to the knees, will be horizontal. Before pushing the body to a horizontal position, the chin should be well down on the chest. Then, as the body is raised, the head should be allowed to drop gently backward as far as it will go. Next, return to a sitting position and relax for a moment before repeating the procedure. When the body is pressed up to the complete horizontal position, tense every muscle in the body. This will have a tendency to stimulate Vortexes 'F,' 'G,' 'E,' 'D' and C.'

"After leaving the Lamasery," continued Colonel Bradford, "I went to a number of the larger cities in India, and as an experiment conducted classes for both English people and natives. I found that the older members of either felt that unless they could perform a Rite perfectly, right from the beginning, they believed no good could come from it. I had considerable difficulty in convincing them that they were wrong. Finally I persuaded them to do the best they could and see just what happened in a month's time. After a good deal of persuasion I was able to get them to do their best, and the results in a month's time were more than gratifying.

"I remember in one city I had quite a number of old people in one of my classes. With this particular Rite – Number Four – they could just barely get their bodies off the floor; they couldn't get it anywhere near a horizontal position. In the same class were several much younger persons who had no difficulty in performing the Rite perfectly from the very start. This so discouraged the older people that I had to ask the younger ones to refrain from practicing it before their older classmates. I explained that I could not do it at first, either; that I couldn't do a bit better than any of them; but that I could perform the Rite 50 times in succession now without feeling the slightest strain on nerves or muscles; and in order to convince them, I did it right before their eyes. From then on, the class broke all records for results accomplished."

(9) *If you don't have sufficient arm strength in the beginning, don't worry—try propping your hands on yoga blocks or folded towels (nothing slippery or uneven like cushions). It will make it easier to lift into the tabletop position. Then, as your arm strength increases, you can cut them in half to reduce the height or remove them altogether.*

RITE NO 4 – THE TABLETOP

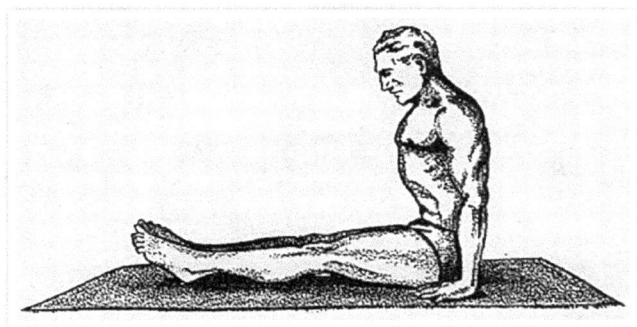

First Position of Rite No. 4

"Sit on the 'prayer rug' with the feet stretched out in front. Then place the hands alongside the body." (*1939 & 1946 Editions – Introduction.*)

"Sit **erect** on **rug or carpet** with feet stretched out in front. **The legs must be perfectly straight – back of knees must be well down or close to the rug. Place the hands flat on the rug, fingers together, and the hands pointing outward slightly. Chin should be on chest – head forward.**" (*1946 Edition – New information is in bold.*)

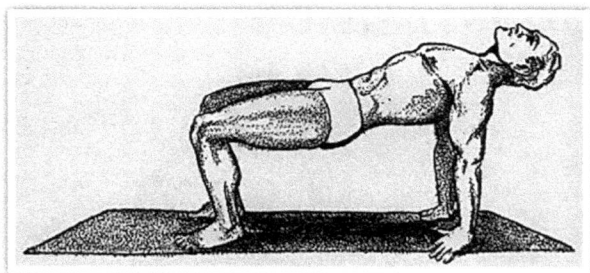

Second Position of Rite No. 4

"Now raise the body and bend the knees so that the legs from the knees down, are practically straight up and down. The arms, too, will be straight up and down while the body, from the shoulders to the knees, will be horizontal. Before pushing the body to a horizontal position the chin should be well down on the chest.

Then, as the body is raised the head should be allowed to drop gently backward as far as it will go.[10] Next, return to a sitting position and relax for a moment before repeating the procedure. When the body is pressed up to the complete horizontal position tense every muscle in the body.[11] This will have the tendency to stimulate Vortexes 'F,' 'G,' 'E,' 'D,' and 'C.'" *(1939 & 1946 Editions – Introduction.)*

> "Now **gently** raise the body, **at the same time** bend the knees so that the legs from the knees down, are practically straight up and down. The arms, too, **will also be vertical** while the body from shoulders to knees will be horizontal.
>
> As the body is raised **upward** allow the head gently to **fall** backward so that the head hangs backward as far as possible **when the body is fully horizontal.**

Hold this position for a few moments, return to first position and RELAX for a few minutes before performing the Rite again." (*1946 Edition – New information is in bold.*)

Energy Breathing

- *Lie on your back, bend your knees and place your hands in the Energy Breathing Position with your hands wrapped around your lower ribs.*

- *Exhale fully, then take three complete Energy Breaths,* **Steps 1, 2,** *or* **3,** *ending with an inhalation (see Chapter 8).*

(10) *For the same reasons as those mentioned in Rite No 3, avoid letting your head "drop gently backward as far as it will go" to prevent compression of your cervical spine and vertebral artery. Instead, keep your head balanced on top of your neck as if you were standing upright.*

(11) ***Tensing All The Muscles.*** *In his new instructions added beneath each illustration in the 1946 update, Kelder left out the sentence, "When the body is pressed up to the complete horizontal position tense every muscle in the body." I mention this because some practitioners believe tensing is significant and perhaps mysterious. But, as you can see from the later 1946 version above, Kelder doesn't attach as much importance to it as they do. A further example of this is Kelder's inconsistency when describing tensing across each Rite. In Rites 2 and 3, Kelder doesn't mention tensing at all, and in Rite 4 he describes the effects of tensing on stimulating the vortexes but omits this instruction for Rite No 5.*

Perhaps Bradford simply means that when we reach the apex of the movement, all our muscles are tensed (which they are) before we move down into the second part of the movement. In practice, it is impossible to avoid having tension in your muscles at these two points in the movement due to the opposing forces of gravity.

Note: *If you suffer from high blood pressure, avoid holding your breath when muscle tensing, as this can raise blood pressure.*

RITE
NUMBER FIVE

"The best way to perform this Rite is to place the hands on the floor about two feet apart. Then, with the legs stretched out to the rear with the feet also about two feet apart, push the body, and especially the hips, up as far as possible, rising on the toes and hands. At the same time the head should be brought so far down that the chin comes up against the chest.

"Next, allow the body to come slowly down to a 'sagging' position. Bring the head up, causing it to be drawn as far back as possible.

"After a few weeks, that is after you become quite proficient in this movement, let the body drop from its highest position to a point almost but not quite touching the floor. The muscles should be tensed for a moment when the body is at the highest point, and again at the lowest point." ["Before the end of the first week this particular Rite will be one of the easiest ones to perform for the average person." – removed from the 1946 update.]

"Everywhere I go," went on the Colonel, "folks, at first, call these Rites physical culture exercises. I would like to make it clearly understood that these are not physical culture exercises at all. They are only performed a few times a day; so few times that they could not possibly be of any value as physical culture movements. What the Rites actually do is this: They start the seven Vortexes spinning at a normal rate of speed; at the speed which is normal for, say, a young, robust, strong, robust, virile man of twenty-five years of age.

"Now in such a person the Vortexes are all spinning normally at the same rate of speed. On the other hand, if you could view the seven Vortexes of the average middle-aged man – weak, unhealthy, and semi-virile, as he is – you would notice at once that some of the Vortexes had greatly slowed down in their spinning movement; and worse still, all were spinning at a different rate of speed – none of them working together in harmony. The slower ones allowed that part of the body which they govern to degenerate, deteriorate, and become diseased." ["The faster ones, spinning at a much greater speed would have caused nervousness and nerve exhaustion. All of them making the individual anything but a real man." – removed from the 1946 update.]

"The only INNER difference between youth and virility, and old age and senility, is simply the difference in the rate of speed at which the Vortexes are spinning. Normalize the different speeds, and the old man becomes a new man again."

RITE NO 5– THE PENDULUM

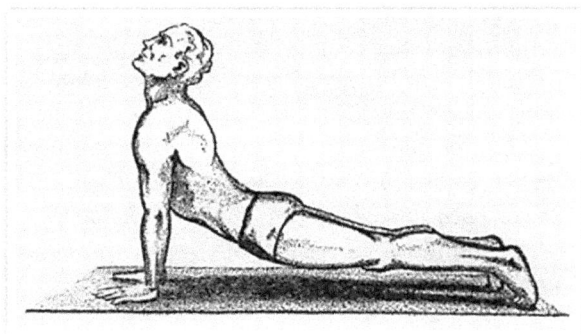

First Position of Rite No. 5

"The best way to perform this Rite[12] is to place the hands on the floor about two feet apart. Then, with the legs stretched out to the rear with the feet also about two feet apart, push the body, and especially the hips, up as far as possible, rising on the toes and hands. At the same time the head should be brought so far down that the chin comes up against the chest.

Next, allow the body to come slowly down to a 'sagging' position. Bring the head up, causing it to be drawn as far back as possible." (*1939 & 1946 Editions – Introduction.*)

"The First position of the Rite is to place the hands on the floor about two feet apart. The legs are stretched out to the rear with the feet also about two feet apart. Allow the body to "sag"[13] **downward from shoulders to toes**. Hold the head as far back as is comfortable. **The arms are kept perfectly straight at all times in Rite No. 5**." (*1946 Edition – New information is in bold.*)

(12) When I began teaching the Rites, I experimented with starting this movement in the upside-down V position. The plank-like position described above requires more physical strength than most beginners can achieve, and it makes no difference to the benefits of this Rites, which way you begin.

Many people prefer this starting position and continue doing it for as long as they practice the Rites. Why don't you try both and see which suits you the best? You can always change back once your strength and flexibility increase.

(13) For the reasons discussed in Rite No 3, avoid 'sagging' in the lower back, as collapsing compresses your vertebrae and discs. Unless you know how to activate your core muscles correctly while maintaining the length in your spine, it is best to avoid overbending. Try gently firming your buttocks instead to prevent you from hollowing out your lower back too much. In the early stages, some people rest their thighs on a bolster for the same reason.

If you want to learn how to identify and engage your core muscles correctly, consider a few Pilates classes or learn from one of the T5T resources listed at the back of this book.

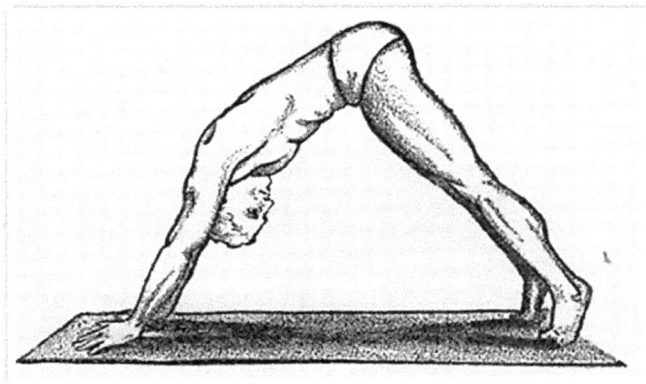

Second Position of Rite No. 5

"After a few weeks, that is after you become quite proficient in this movement, let the body drop from its highest position to a point almost but not quite touching the floor. The muscles should be tensed for a moment when the body is at the highest point, and again at the lowest point." *(1939 & 1946 Editions – Introduction.)* ["Before the end of the first week this particular Rite will be one of the easiest ones to perform for the average person." – removed from the 1946 update.]

"The Second position is attained by pushing the body, especially the hips, upward as far as possible. The hands are kept flat on the floor at all times. Hold this position for a brief moment and return to First position. After a moment of "hanging in suspension" perform the Rite over again." *(1946 Edition – New information is in bold.)*

Note: *As you can see, this entire description is new and is Kelder's biggest edit so far. It is also significant in that, once again, he doesn't mention muscle tensing– he merely says, "Hold this position for a brief moment."*

Energy Breathing

- *When you have finished your repetitions, simply bend your knees and drop them to the floor so that you are back on your hands and knees. Come into Child's Pose and move your knees slightly apart to prepare for Energy Breathing. As you breathe, focus on the muscles of your back – expanding and contracting.*

- *Begin by exhaling fully, then take three complete Energy Breaths, **Steps 1, 2,** or **3,** ending with an inhalation (see Chapter 8). If you have time, you can carry out one of the breathing-based meditations in Chapter 9.*

FURTHER INFORMATION

When the Colonel had finished his description of the Five Rites I said to him,

"Let me ask you some questions now."

"Very well," he replied. "That is just what I want you to do."

"I feel that from your description I understand the Rites quite well," I began, "but when and how often are they to be employed?"

"They can be used either night and morning," answered the Colonel, "in the morning only, or just at night, if it is more convenient. I use them both morning and night, but I would not advise so much stimulation for the beginner until he has practiced them for a number of months. At the start he could use them the full number of times in the morning, and then in the evening he could gradually build up until finally he is doing the same amount of practice as in the morning."

"Just how many times a day should a person use these Rites?" was my next question.

"To start with," said he, "I would suggest you practice each Rite three times a day for the first week. Then increase them by two a day each week until you are doing 21 a day; which will be at the beginning of the 10th week."[14]

(14) Everyone wants to reach the goal of 21 repetitions – some as quickly as possible. However, there is a lot to be gained by building up repetitions exactly as described by Kelder (3 reps in your first week, adding 2 per week until you are doing 21 in ten weeks' time.) We humans are always rushing towards some future experience, and you would benefit significantly from slowing down and being present to your experiences when learning the Rites. Arriving at your destination of 21 repetitions will be all the more fulfilling if you do so.

People who practice yoga regularly or keep themselves fit may want to progress at a much faster rate than Colonel Bradford recommends. This is understandable, but please remember that these exercises are designed to have a stimulating effect on the energy systems of your body. If, after having performed the Rites, you find it difficult to relax or remain focused, are moodier than usual, have difficulty sleeping, or feel you are "not in" your body – then reduce repetitions and build up more gradually.

If you feel slightly nauseous or have a mild headache, then you are doing too many repetitions – most likely due to the spinning movement of the 1st Rite. See Appendix (A), at the back of the book for more information on dizziness.

DETOX EFFECTS

Due to the increased elimination of impurities and wastes and elevated oxygen levels in your body, you may experience some minor detox effects. Some people have strong changes, and others have none at all. If you do experience any of the following symptoms, they usually settle down within a week.

A metallic taste in the mouth.

Achy joints for a day or so.

Darker, stronger-smelling urine.

Diarrhoea or a strong bowel movement.

Initial constipation.

Slight nausea.

Initial fatigue as the body balances itself.

Cold or flu-like symptoms that last a day.

A runny nose as sinuses clear.

A tic or involuntary muscle movement over one eye.
A mild rash or pimples.

Moodiness, either a bit snappy or teary.

FURTHER INFORMATION - CONTINUED

"If you cannot practice Rite Number One, the whirling one, the same number of times as the others, then do it only as many times as you can without getting too dizzy. The time will soon come, however, when you can practice it the full number of 21 times."

["I knew of one man who required more than a year before he could do it that many times. But he performed the other four without difficulty, gradually increasing the number until he was doing the full 21 on all four. He got very splendid results.

"Under certain conditions," added the Colonel, "there are some who find it difficult to perform Rite Number One at all, to begin with. But after having done the other four for about six months they are amazed at how easy it is to do Number

One. Likewise with the other Rites." - *removed from the 1946 update*.] If for any reason one or more of them cannot be used, do not be discouraged; use what you can. Results, in that case, will be a little slower, but that is the only handicap.

"If one has been recently operated on for, say, appendicitis, or is afflicted with hernia, he should be very cautious in practicing Rites Numbers Two, Three, and Five. If one is very heavy, he should be cautious in the use of Number Five until his weight has been greatly reduced.

"All five of the Rites are of importance. Even though he may not be able to perform them the prescribed number of times the individual may rest assured that just a few times each day will be of benefit.

"If, at the end of the fourth week, one finds that he cannot perform every one of the Rites the required number of times, he should note carefully the ones which he is forced to slight. Then, if he is performing the Five Rites in the morning, he should try to make up the deficiency in the evening. Or if he is performing the Rites in the evening, he should endeavor to find time in the morning to catch up. In either event he should not neglect the other Rites, and above all he should never strain himself. If he goes about performing the Rites in an easy, interesting manner it will not be long before he finds everything working out satisfactorily, and that he is doing the Rites the required 21 times a day.

"Some people, acting on their own initiative, invent little aids for their practices. An old fellow in India found it impossible for him to perform Rite Number Four properly even once. He wouldn't be satisfied with just getting his body off the floor; he was determined that it should reach a horizontal position as the Rite prescribed. So he got a box about ten inches high and two and a half feet long. Upon this he put some bedding folded to the right size, and across this padded box he lay flat on his back. Then, with his feet on the floor at one end and his hands on the floor at the other he found it quite simple to raise his body to a horizontal position.

"Now while this little 'stunt' may not in itself have helped the old gentleman in performing the Rite the full 21 times, still the psychological effect of being able to raise his body as high as the much stronger men was undoubtedly quite stimulating and may have been quite beneficial. I do not particularly recommend this old man's aid, although it may help those who think it impossible to make progress in any other way; but if you have an inventive mind you will think of ways and means to help you in performing the more difficult Rites.

"These Rites are so powerful that if one were left out entirely while the other four were practiced regularly the full number of times, only the finest kind of results would be experienced. Only one Rite alone [The 1946 update says, "The First Rite"] will do wonders, as evidenced by the Whirling Dervishes of whom we spoke. Had they spun around only a limited number of times, they would have found themselves greatly benefited, although they may not have attributed their improved condition to the whirling. The fact that they whirled from left to right[15] and that the old men, who no doubt whirled around less than the younger ones, were virile and strong is ample proof that just one Rite will have powerful effects. "So if anyone finds that they simply cannot perform all five of these practices, or that they cannot perform them all the full number of times, they may still know that good results may still be experienced from what they were able to do."

> (15) *As mentioned earlier in the description for Rite No 1, this information is incorrect: The Dervishes spin anti-clockwise – from right to left.*

"Does anything else go with these Five Rites?" I asked.

"There are two more things which would help. The first is to stand erect with hands on hips between the Five Rites and take one or two deep breaths. [**Note: The 1946 Edition completely excludes this information on breathing.**] The other suggestion is to take either a tepid bath or a cool, but not cold, one after practicing the Rites. Going over the body quickly with a wet towel and then with a dry one is probably even better. One thing I must caution you against: you must never take a shower, tub, or wet towel bath which is cold enough to chill you even slightly internally. If you do, you will have undone all the good you have gained from performing the Five Rites."

"This all seems so simple," I ventured, "do you mean to tell me that this is all that is necessary in the work of restoring the senile, [1946 Edition says "prematurely"] old men to robust health, vigor, and virility?"

"All that is required," answered the Colonel, "is to practice the Five Rites three times a day to begin with, and gradually increase them as I have explained until each is being practiced 21 times each day. That is all; there is nothing more.

"Of course," he continued, "one must practice them every day in order to keep one's robust vitality. You may skip one day a week, but never more than that. The use of the Five Rites is no hardship at all; it requires less than 10 minutes a day to practice them. If necessary one can get up ten minutes earlier or go to bed ten minutes later.

"The Five Rites are for the express purpose of restoring a man to manhood. That is, to make him virile and keep him that way constantly. Whether or not he will make the come-back in youthful appearance, as I have done in so short a time, depends on how he uses his virility. Some men do not care whether they look young, or even whether they appear young, just so long as they have all their manly powers. But as for me, I was an old man for so many years, practically forty, that I like the idea of throwing off the years in every way possible."

16

THE FIVE ELEMENTS

At the time of the development of the Five Tibetan Rites of Rejuvenation, the ancients believed that their world was composed of Five Elements: water, earth, air, fire, and spirit (energy).

In psychology, the Five Elements are used to personify different human traits, such as the personality type categories of Carl Jung (feeling, sensing, intuiting, and thinking) and those associated with the astrological signs of the zodiac. I experimented with the concept of adding an element and an affirmation to each of the Rites. Many people have found the results to be amazing. You can try them and see if they work as well for you.

In each case, the physical movement of the Rite was a metaphor for what we were trying to achieve mentally – awareness of a different aspect of life. For example, the Spin takes the element energy, and the vortex that the movements create allows you to replenish your body from the larger energy all around us. The Tabletop takes the element earth, and its movements focus on stability, foundation, and balance, giving us a solid base from which to form new ideas.

In holistic exercise, it can sometimes be hard to marry the physical state with the mental state, and having a metaphor helps people align the two and present a clear picture of what they are working towards.

Having assigned an element and a modern name to each Rite, I then experimented with creating an affirmation that expressed the "energy" of each movement. The result is a method of reinforcing and focusing on the positive benefits of each Rite physically, mentally, and spiritually. This has a ripple effect on every area of your life.

- **Rite No. I (Energy)**
  – The Spin – "I am full of energy."
- **Rite No. 2 (Air)**
  – The Leg Raise – "My mind is clear and calm."
- **Rite No. 3 (Water)**
  – The Kneeling Backbend – "I am flexible and receptive."
- **Rite No. 4 (Earth)**
  – The Tabletop – "I am strong and balanced."
- **Rite No. 5 (Fire)**
  – The Pendulum – "I am positive and motivated."

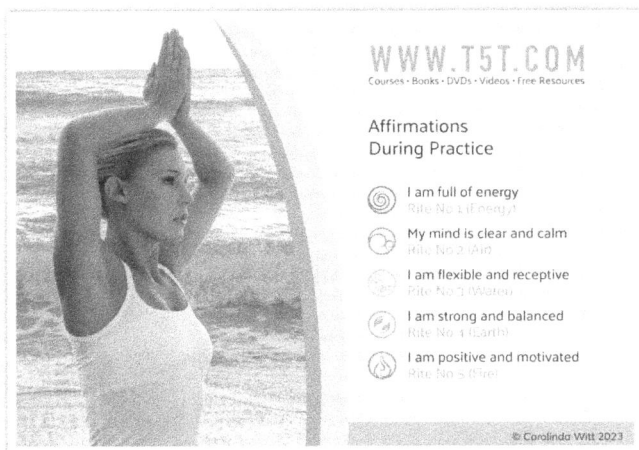

You can download this free Affirmations Poster on the *T5T. com* website.

17

THE HIMALAYA CLUB

It had been ten weeks since Colonel Bradford's return from India. Much had happened in that time. I had immediately started putting the Five Rites into practice and had been getting most gratifying results. The Colonel had been busy with some personal business transactions and I saw little of him for a while, but when he once more was at leisure I lost no time telling him of my progress and in enthusiastically expressing my feeling regarding this wonderful new system of regaining health, vigor, power, virility, and vitality.

Ever since the day I was sure that I was well on the way to new youth and vigor, I had been thinking what a splendid idea it would be to pass on the information about the Five Rites to my friends, and now that the Colonel had time to spare I approached him with the idea of forming a class. He agreed that it was a very commendable idea and agreed to teach it himself on three conditions.

The first of these conditions was that the class should comprise a cross-section of men from all walks of life-from ditch-diggers to bankers. The second condition was that no member could be under 50 years of age, although they could be up to a hundred or more, if I knew anyone that old. These two conditions met with my satisfaction; but the third was a big disappointment. The Colonel insisted that the class be limited to 15 members, and I had ten times that number in mind. However, no amount of persuasion and coercion could change his mind.

From the beginning the class was a huge success. We met once a week and my friends all had implicit faith in the Colonel and in the Five Rites. As early as the second week I could see marked improvement in several of them, although, being forbidden to discuss their progress with anyone but the Colonel, I could not verify my impression. However, at the end of a month we held a kind of testimonial meeting. Every man reported improvement. Some told most glowing accounts. A man nearing 75 years of age had made more gains than any of the others.

The weekly meetings of "The Himalaya Club," as we had named it, continued. The tenth week rolled around and practically all of the members were performing all Five Rites 21 times a day. All of them were feeling better and some dropped a number of years from their appearance and jokingly gave their ages as younger than they really were. This brought to mind that several of them had asked the Colonel his age but that he had told them he would wait until the end of the tenth week to tell them. This was the evening, but as yet the Colonel had not put in an appearance. Some one suggested that each member write on a slip of paper what age he believed the Colonel to be and then they would compare notes. As the papers were being collected, in walked Colonel Bradford. When he was told what had taken place he said.

"Bring them to me and I shall see how well you have estimated my age. Then I shall tell you what it really is."

The slips all read from 38 to 42. With great amusement the Colonel read them aloud.

"Gentlemen," he said, "I thank you. You are most complimentary. And as you have been honest with me, I shall be equally honest with you. I shall be 73 years of age on my next birthday."

The members stared in consternation and amazement. They found it hard to believe that one so youthful in appearance could have lived so long. Then they wanted to know why, inasmuch as they already felt half their former age, they, too, had not made more progress in youthful appearance.

"In the first place, gentlemen," the Colonel informed them, "you have only been doing this wonderful work for ten weeks. When you have been at it two years you will see a much more pronounced change. Then again, I have not told you all there is to know. I have given you five Rites which are for the express purpose of restoring one to manly vigor and vitality. These Five Rites also make one appear more youthful; but if you really want to look and be young in every respect there is a Sixth Rite that you must practice. I have said nothing about it until now because it would have been useless to you without first having obtained good results from the other five."

The Colonel then informed them that in order to go further with the aid of this Sixth Rite it would be necessary for them to lead a more or less continent life.[16] He suggested that they take a week to think the matter over and decide whether or not they desired to do so for the rest of their lives. Then those who wished to go on would be given Rite Number Six. There were but five who came back the next week, although according to the Colonel this was a better showing than he had experienced with any of his classes in India.

(16) More or less 'continent' means more or less celibate (abstinence from sexual intercourse.)

When he had first told them about the Sixth Rite, the Colonel had made it clear that the procreative energy would be lifted up, and that this lifting-up process would cause not only the mind to be renewed but the entire body as well; but that it entailed certain restrictions with which the average man[17] did not care to conform. Then he went on with this explanation.

> (17) *Although Kelder did not provide any instructions for women, possibly because the monastery only contained men, many thousands of women worldwide have successfully practiced the Rites and obtained the same great benefits as men.*
>
> *It is important to acknowledge that the majority of practitioners, regardless of gender, only practice the Five Rites, and these five exercises alone are sufficient to obtain the great benefits described in this book.*

"In the average virile man," said the Colonel, "the life forces course downward, but in order to become a Super-man they must be turned upward. This we call 'The Newer Use of the Reproductive Energy.' Turning these powerful forces upward is a very simple matter, yet man has attempted it in many ways for centuries and in almost every instance has failed. Whole religious orders in the Occidental World have tried this very thing, but they, too, have failed because they have tried to master the procreative energy by suppressing it. There is only one way to master this powerful urge, and that is not by dissipating or suppressing it but by TRANSMUTING it – transmuting it and at the same time lifting it upward. In this way you really and truly have discovered not only the 'Elixir of Life,' as the ancients called it, but you have put it to use as well, which is something the ancients were seldom able to do.

"Now this Rite Number Six is the simplest thing in the world to perform. It should only be practiced when one has an excess of procreative energy; when there is a definite desire for expression. It can be done so easily that it can be performed anywhere at any time. When one feels the powerful reproductive urge, here is all that is necessary:

"Stand erect and then let all the air out of the lungs, as one bends over and places his hands on his knees. Force out the last trace of air. Then, with empty lungs, stand erect, place hands on hips, and push down on them. This has a tendency to push up the shoulders. While doing this, pull in the abdomen just as far as possible, which raises the chest. Now hold this position as long as you can. Then when you are forced to take air into the empty lungs, let the air flow in through the nose. Exhale it through the mouth as you relax the arms and let them hang naturally at your sides. Then take several deep breaths through the mouth or nose and allow them to quickly escape through either the mouth or the nose. This constitutes one complete performance of Rite Number Six[18]. About three are required to subdue the most powerful urge and to turn the powerful procreative or reproductive forces upward.

> (18) Interestingly, the Sixth Rite is similar to a yoga practice known as 'Uddiyana Bandha,' which means 'flying upward energy lock.' It is one of three bandhas (energy locks or valves) that are practiced together or individually at specific times during yoga postures, breathing, visualization, meditation, and other yogic practices.
>
> The bandhas direct energy (prana) throughout the body to release blockages and nourish corresponding areas. They bind or 'lock' the prana to prevent it from dissipating from the body. Bandhas, when released, allow the flow of

kundalini energy up the central energy canal in the spinal column, which connects the base chakra to the crown chakra.

"The only difference there is between the average virile man and the Super-man is that the virile lets the procreative urge flow downward while the Super-man turns the procreative urge upward and reproduces within himself a new-man – a strong, powerful, magnetic man who is constantly growing younger, day by day, moment by moment. This is the true SUPER-MAN, who creates within himself the true 'ELIXIR OF LIFE.' Now you understand why it was unnecessary for me to have left my native England to find the 'Fountain of Youth'– it was within me all the time. Now you can see that when I wrote you some time ago that I had found 'The Fountain of Youth' and was bringing it back with me, I meant just that. The Five Rites and the 'Fountain' are one.

"When I remember Ponce de Leon and his futile search for the 'Fountain' I think of how simple it would have been for him to stay at home and simply use it; but he, like myself, believed it was anywhere in the world except within one's self.

"Please understand that in order to perform Rite Number Six it is absolutely necessary that a man have full masculine virility. He couldn't possibly raise up and transmute procreative energy if there were little or none to transmute. It is absolutely impossible for an impotent man or the one with little virility to perform this Rite. He shouldn't even attempt it, because it would only lead to discouragement, which might do him great harm. Instead he should first practice the other five Rites until he has full masculine power, and this regardless of how young or how old he may be. Then when the first full bloom of youth is experienced within him, he may, if he wishes, go on to the business of being a SUPER-MAN.

"The man of the world is interested only in the material things of the world, and for that reason should practice only the first five Rites until he feels the urge or desire within to become the SUPER-MAN. Then he should decide definitely; for a clean-cut start and a new life are absolutely necessary to those who lead the SUPER-LIFE. They are the ones who become MYSTICS, OCCULTISTS, and ADEPTS. They it is who truly see with THE EYE OF REVELATION.

"Again I say, let no man concern himself with the up-turning of the sex currents until he is thoroughly satisfied in his own mind and heart that he truly desires to lead the life of the MYSTIC; then let him make the step forward, and success will crown his every effort."

RITE
NUMBER SIX

From my experience, people who are interested in practicing the Sixth Rite generally fall into two camps. The first will try it and see what happens, and the second will carry out further research, such as reading tantric texts or obtaining instruction from recognized tantric teachers.

According to author and scholar, Dr. Peter Baofu, "the tantric practitioner seeks to use the prana (divine power) that flows through the universe (including one's own body) to attain purposeful goals. These goals may be spiritual, material, or both. Most practitioners of tantra consider mystical experience imperative. Some versions of Tantra require the guidance of a guru."

In the process of working with energy, the tantric practitioner has various tools at hand: Yoga, visualizations, yantras, mantras, mudras, meditation, mind training, identification & internalization of deities, mandalas, feasts, purification achievements, initiations, and more.

"Secrecy protects the tantric practitioner and his practice in several ways. It is said that the power and efficacy of the Vajrayana is dependent upon the devotion and respect of its practitioners. If one were to disclose to non-initiates one's practices and experiences, these would be met with misunderstanding and lack of appreciation, at the very least."

—**Reginald A Ray,** *Secret of the Vajra World: The Tantric Buddhism of Tibet.*

The 6th Rite is similar to Uddiyana Bandha, a Hatha yoga exercise commonly practiced by men and women. Both versions are included below.

HERE ARE KELDER'S INSTRUCTIONS ON HOW TO DO THE SIXTH RITE:

- *Stand erect and then let all the air out of the lungs, as one bends over and places his hands on his knees. Force out the last trace of air.*

- *Then, with empty lungs, stand erect, place hands on hips, and push down on them. This has a tendency to push up the shoulders.*

- *While doing this, pull in the abdomen just as far as possible, which raises the chest. Now hold this position as long as you can.*

- *Then when you are forced to take air into the empty lungs, let the air flow in through the nose.*

- *Exhale it through the mouth as you relax the arms and let them hang naturally at your sides.*

- *Then take several deep breaths through the mouth or nose and allow them to quickly escape through either the mouth or the nose.*

- *This constitutes one complete performance of Rite Number Six. About three are required to subdue the most powerful urge and to turn the powerful procreative or reproductive forces upward.*

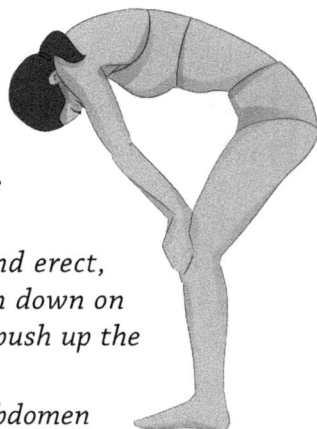

UDDIYANA BANDHA INSTRUCTIONS

In Hatha yoga it is recommended that you should only carry out uddiyana bandha on an empty stomach as the abdomen is contracted, up, and into the rib cage. It is performed only after an exhalation and never before an inhalation.

❑ *Stand with your feet slightly apart and your knees bent.*

❑ *Round your torso forward with your hands resting on your knees.*

❑ *Inhale deeply, then exhale forcibly and quickly through your nose or mouth.*

❑ *Pull in (contract) your belly muscles to force as much air as possible out of your lungs.*

❑ *Relax your abdominals and expand your rib cage as though you were inhaling (but without the inhalation) – often called a "mock inhalation." This hollows the stomach, pulling it in and up towards the rib cage.*

❑ *Hold the bandha for about 5 – 15 seconds, then slowly release the grip and inhale normally.*

❑ *Between each repetition—around 3 to 10, depending on your capacity, take a few normal breaths.*

19

CHOOSING THE RIGHT METHOD FOR YOU

F it or not, I recommend you follow Colonel Bradford's advice by beginning with three repetitions (of each Rite) per day in your first week. Then, every week, add two more repetitions of each Rite like this –

Week One - 3 reps per day of Rites 1-5

Week Two – 5 reps per day of Rites 1-5

Week Three – 7 reps per day of Rites 1-5

Week Four – 9 reps per day of Rites 1-5

Week Five – 11 reps per day and so on

Following the monks' instructions, you will reach the required 21 repetitions in ten weeks. This may seem like a long time to get to 21, but I can assure you the arrival at your destination will be all the richer for having undergone the journey to get there.

Your body needs time to adjust to changes to your balance system and energy system. Building up repetitions too quickly can create a detox effect as well as a degree of dizziness or nausea. These side effects can be improved or avoided altogether by gradually increasing your repetitions.

Remember this isn't just physical exercise – the true purpose of the Rites as described by Kelder is:

"The body has seven centers, which, in English, could be called Vortexes. These are kind of magnetic centers. They revolve at great speed in the healthy body, but when slowed down – well that is just another name for old age, ill-health, and senility. These spinning centers of activity extend beyond the flesh in the healthy individual, but in the old, weak, senile person they hardly reach the surface, except in the knees. The quickest way to regain health, youth, and vitality is to start these magnetic centers spinning again. There are but five practices that will do this. Any one of them will be helpful, but all five are required to get glowing results. These five exercises are really not exercises at all, in the physical culture sense. The Lamas think of them as 'Rites' and so instead of calling them exercises or practices, we too, shall call them 'Rites'."

—**Peter Kelder,** *The Eye of Revelation.*

LEARNING THE RITES

Throughout these pages, I have shared some of my knowledge about teaching The Five Tibetan Rites for the past twenty-three years. However, this book was never intended to be a complete instructional manual—its purpose was to share Peter Kelder's unadulterated words and some valuable tips.

Naturally, there is a lot more I can share with you, but for now, here is a brief overview of what I have learned in case you want to know more.

The reason I call the Rites "T5T" is because it is a lot quicker than saying "The Five Tibetan Rites." Having spent so many years fine-honing a method of learning the Rites that is unique in its methods, there needed to be a way of identifying it from everyone else. Also, the T5T method produces additional benefits.

Through its step-by-step learning method and focus on core strength development, T5T enables practitioners to increase their core stability to protect and support their spines. Practitioners also practice breathing techniques with and between each Rite, which improves their breathing capacity. Importantly, the benefits received are exactly the same as those described by Kelder in his books.

Most people will find the descriptions in this book sufficient to learn the Rites, particularly if they are younger and fitter, have good body-mind awareness, and have not suffered from a back or neck injury in the past.

Since the Five Tibetan Rites are repetitive movements, there are some key points to be aware of to avoid strain or injury, particularly if you want to establish a long-term practice. T5T is a method of learning the Rites that has been tried and tested by thousands of students worldwide and is ideal for anyone who wants more in-depth instructions than the simple ones provided by Kelder.

It is an ideal way of learning the Rites for anyone wishing to learn how to move their body safely while carrying out these movements daily—and is particularly helpful for those needing modifications or adaptations due to muscle weakness or injury.

Most of all, T5T is for those who want to protect and strengthen their bodies' vulnerable areas—their lower backs and necks—not just when performing the Rites but also in everyday life.

Consider this: When you have built up to 21 repetitions of each movement (five postures performed 21 times each), you will be doing 105 repetitions per day. Over a year (365 days), that is 38,325 repetitions. As you can imagine, it is vital to have correct alignment and technique.

One of the principal things we have learned from fine-tuning solutions to solve students' common problems is the importance of developing strong core muscles to protect the spine. It is also the key to a successful long-term practice and a short-term pleasurable learning experience.

- *Core muscles are the deepest muscles closest to the spine, and when correctly activated, they wrap around and protect the spine like a natural weight belt or girdle.*

  (a) *The first step is learning to correctly identify and activate your core muscles. It is easy to use the stronger, more external muscles of the abdomen instead, leaving the inner muscles underdeveloped (like a soft-centered chocolate.)*

  (b) *To achieve core strength, we follow the 10-week build-up recommendations of the monks mentioned earlier but include a variation in how we do the 2nd Rite (the Leg Raise) every week.*

  (c) *Just like lifting weights at the gym: You begin with low loads (in our case, the natural weight of the legs) and gradually increase the load and repetitions by shifting from single-leg to double-leg movements or from bent legs to straight legs.*

- *As you have read, T5T incorporates **natural full breathing** when practicing the Rites (and between each Rite) due to the great benefits optimal breathing provides to vitality and health.*

- *For people who cannot do the Rites exactly as described, we provide **modifications** that do not reduce the benefits of the Rites in any way.*

"**T5T** is an incredible and powerful program. It turns back the clock. It increases your energy, mental clarity, and focus. It reduces stress and improves strength and flexibility. It is capable of restoring your passion and zest for life if you let it. I highly recommend it for anyone willing to improve their life."

—John Gray ~
Author of *Men are from Mars, Women are from Venus*

THINGS TO BE CONSIDERED BEFORE LEARNING THE RITES

Are you currently doing very little exercise?	*YES/NO*
Have you ever practiced yoga before?	*YES/NO*
Have you suffered from back pain or neck pain in the past?	*YES/NO*
Have you seen any therapist for back or neck pain in the past?	*YES/NO*
Is one side of your body (or one limb) noticeably stronger than the other?	*YES/NO*
Have you noticed any muscular weakness in any part of your body?	*YES/NO*
Have you noticed any stiffness in any part of your body?	*YES/NO*
Do you find it an effort to maintain an upright stance when sitting or standing? Do you slouch?	*YES/NO*
Do you hold tension in your shoulders and upper back?	*YES/NO*
Do you have weak or inflexible wrists? Do you find it a bit of a struggle to unscrew jars/bottles etc.?	*YES/NO*
Do you find it difficult to turn your neck around sufficiently when reversing your car?	*YES/NO*
Are you overweight?	*YES/NO*
Are you largely sedentary? Do you spend most of your time sitting in front of a desk or relaxing at home?	*YES/NO*
Are you at a point where you think you had better 'do' something now, before it is too late?	*YES/NO*

DO YOU HAVE MORE YES ANSWERS THAN NO?

Are You Fit Or Relatively Fit?

Would you describe your level of fitness as being good across all four levels below?

Muscle tone	☐
Flexibility & range of motion	☐
Body awareness	☐
Energy & stamina	☐

Is core stability part of your workout?   YES/NO

Are you able to identify and isolate each core muscle; the pelvic floor, transversus abdominis & multifidus muscles.   YES/NO

Do you know when or if you incorrectly use your obliques to stabilise rather than your core muscles?   YES/NO

Do you know how to establish and maintain neutral spine and neutral pelvis, whilst keeping your head and neck in line with your spine?   YES/NO

How good is your breathing? If you already practice pranayama, are you also aware of what natural, full breathing should feel like. Consider this:
a. *Are all your breathing spaces able to open when breathing fully? Wide to the side, the back, the front, the ribs?*   YES/NO
b. *Do you have tension/tightness in your breathing?*
c. *How are your stress levels? Do you find yourself breathing rapidly into the upper chest, holding your breath, yawning or sighing?*

Having completed this questionnaire, you should have a better idea of which method of learning the Five Tibetan Rites is best for you. Many people begin practicing by following the instructions in this book. If you start this way and discover you need more detailed explanations and alternatives, swapping to the T5T method is easy. Please see the resources at the back of the book.

Regardless of which method you use, you will find loads of answers to frequently asked questions, resources, information, and interesting articles on my T5T website.

If you would like to join a group of fellow practitioners on Facebook, or connect with the author – see details at the back of the book.

AFTERWORD

The Tibetan way of life today is unrecognizable from the one 'Colonel Bradford' described in 1939. Just ten years later, in 1949, Mao Zedong proclaimed the founding of the People's Republic of China and threatened to 'liberate' Tibet. In 1951 Tibetan leaders were forced to sign a treaty agreeing to the establishment of Chinese civil and military headquarters in Lhasa, but mounting resentment against Chinese rule led to armed resistance, leading to a full-scale uprising in Lhasa in 1959. During the suppression of the revolt, where thousands are said to have died, the Dalai Lama, most of his ministers, and around 80,000 other Tibetans fled to Dharamsala in India, where they have remained ever since.

According to the Tibetan Government in Exile, an estimated 1.2 million Tibetans have died as a direct result of Chinese occupation, and over 6,000 monasteries, temples and countless sacred texts and religious artifacts have been destroyed.

If you want to know more or want to help support Tibetan charities, please visit the *website* of the Central Tibetan Administration (CTA), where the Tibetan people, under the leadership of His Holiness the Dalai Lama, have been carrying out a non-violent movement to regain their lost freedom and dignity.

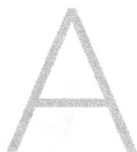

A IMPROVE YOUR SPIN TECHNIQUE TO REDUCE DIZZINESS AND NAUSEA

1. **Slow Down.** *Don't try and complete too many rotations too quickly. Allow your body time to get used to the motion.*

2. **Do Fewer Repetitions.** *Some people take six months or more to build up to the required 21 repetitions. Dizziness affects people differently regardless of their fitness level. I have taught yoga teachers & long-term yoga practitioners who experienced dizziness in the early stages of learning the Spin. Do only as many repetitions as you can without becoming uncomfortably dizzy. Gradually add repetitions over a period of weeks or even months until you can do the required 21 repetitions easily. Ensure all dizziness has disappeared (to prevent nausea) before moving onto Rite No. 2.*

3. **Continue To Build Repetitions Of Rites, 2, 3, 4, and 5** *in the recommended manner (3 repetitions in your first week, then add 2 per week until you are doing 21 repetitions in around ten weeks). Gradually increase the number of spins until you catch up with the other Rites.*

4. **Fine Tune Your Movement.** *Fine-tune your movement so it is smooth from head to toe. Steps that are too large, too small, too bouncy, or steps that start and stop instead of flowing from one to another create a motion of their own*

and contribute to dizziness. A smooth movement improves aerodynamics and reduces motion.

5. **Flat And Solid Level Surface.** *Do not spin on an uneven surface as this increases dizziness, and you will find it hard to keep your balance. Doing the Rites outside in nature is wonderful, but choose your surface carefully. Soft sand isn't suitable if you are going to try it on a beach.*

6. **Important – Keep Your Spin Movement Contained Within A Small, Obstacle Free Area.** *If you wander across the floor, slow down and adjust your movement. Bring your legs to hip-width apart and take small (not jerky) flowing steps. If you come into contact with an obstacle, avoid looking at it until you have stopped spinning and your dizziness has abated. Otherwise, you will feel very dizzy and may stagger or fall. In T5T, we carry out three special Energy Breaths after spinning. We place our hands on our hips and keep our eyes closed. You could try taking three deep, slow breaths instead.*

7. **Remember to Breathe!** *People often hold their breath while spinning, which reduces the oxygen supply to the brain and increases the likelihood of dizziness. Get into a habit of taking a breath before you begin spinning and constantly remind yourself to breathe normally while performing the Spin.*

ABOUT THE AUTHOR

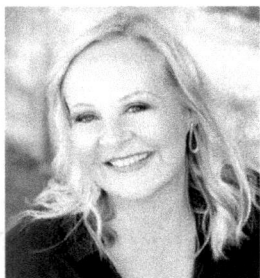

Carolinda Witt is an award-winning author who lives in Sydney.

She keeps herself fit and healthy by practicing The Five Tibetan Rites, which she began in 2000. Carolinda has taught the Rites to over 70,000 people worldwide through her books, online training course, DVD, and workshops – and attributes them to her youthful appearance and energetic outlook.

Carolinda highly recommends the Five Rites to anyone seeking a quick, easy, and effective daily exercise routine.

OTHER BOOKS, VIDEOS & ONLINE TRAINING COURSES BY THIS AUTHOR

Visit your favorite online retailer or the *T5T.com* website to discover other items by Carolinda Witt.

1) **ONLINE TRAINING COURSE**
   - *Five Tibetan Rites Masterclass - Workbook & Video Series*

2) **PAPERBACK & EBOOKS**
   1. *The Five Tibetans Breathing Book* – (UnMind Pty Ltd)
   2. *The Illustrated Five Tibetan Rites* – (UnMind Pty Ltd)
   3. *The Eye of Revelation* – (UnMind Pty Ltd)

3) **DVD**
   - *The Five Tibetans DVD Plus 2 x Bonus Training Manuals (PDF)* – UnMind Pty Ltd

4) **LATEST BOOK**
   - *Double Agent Celery: MI5's Crooked Hero* – (Pen & Sword Books, UK)

Carolinda's grandfather, Walter Dicketts, an ex-RNAS officer, was recruited by MI5 and sent into Nazi Germany to infiltrate the German Secret Service in the guise of a traitor. If Dicketts succeeded, he was to extract crucial secrets about Germany's plans to invade Britain and communicate them back to MI5. With his life on the line, Dicketts managed to outwit his interrogators in Hamburg and Berlin before returning to Britain as, in the Nazi's eyes, a German spy. He didn't realize he had been betrayed before he even entered Germany.

Her grandfather married six times (two of them were mistresses). He had six children to four different wives, most of whom knew nothing about the other and, in Carolinda's mother's case – about Dicketts himself. Sadly, Carolinda's mother died without ever knowing his name. Unable to tell her mother, Carolinda spent seven years researching and writing this book in her memory. What she discovered about Dicketts changed history and reunited a family.

- Non-fiction prize 2018 – Society of Women Writers
- *Wall Street Journal: "Five Best Books About Clandestine Agents in WW11"*

Please consider rating or reviewing this book on *Amazon*, *Goodreads* or other retailer. It will help others learn about the benefits of a regular Five Tibetans practice. Thank you.

FURTHER BREATHING RESOURCES

Most people find combining breathing with their daily Five Tibetans practice is all they need. However, if you wish to study other breathing courses, I recommend you establish a strong daily practice before you do so.

When you introduce too many new things at once, it can be hard to tell which one is driving any changes. Evaluating each practice individually can help you decide which to keep in your daily life and which to let go.

Here are some connections I've found helpful—feel free to explore and discover what works best for you.

1) Book - ***Breath - The New Science Of A Lost Art*** - James Nestor's bestselling book on breathing can be read at anytime and I am sure you will find it interesting.

2) Optimal Breathing - Michael Grant White
   - ***Optimal Breathing Self Mastery Kit*** - Mike's advanced and versatile natural breathing development program.
   - ***Breathing Test*** - Provides an assessment of various aspects of your breathing, including measurements, abilities, and qualities.

- ***Articles*** - Free access to a vast collection of articles and research on breathing.

3) Oxygen Advantage - Buteyko Breathing Method - Patrick McKeown
   - ***Training Course Options***
   - ***Free Breathing App***

4) Conscious Breathing - Anders Olsson
   - ***Conscious Breathing Foundation Course***

5) MyoTape - Mouth tapes that surround the mouth, encouraging nasal breathing without covering the lips. *https://myotape.com/*

CONNECT WITH CAROLINDA WITT

I really appreciate you reading my book! Here are my social media coordinates:

1. *Connect with other Five Tibetans practitioners and me on my Facebook group – fivetibetanritesofrejuvenation*

2. *Visit my websites: www.t5t.com and carolindawitt.com*

3. *Visit my T5T blog and FAQ which has loads of interesting articles and information about practicing the Five Tibetan Rites and includes the latest research.*

ENDNOTES

Chapter 1 – Stop the Clock.

1. Kelder, Peter, *The Eye of Revelation, 1939* Edition, page 5.

2. 6000 Tibetan Monasteries destroyed. *https://www.gatestoneinstitute.org/15413/china-tibet-dialogue*

3. Lopez, Donald S. *"Buddha." Encyclopedia Britannica*, 24 Mar. 2024, *https://www.britannica.com/biography/Buddha-founder-of-Buddhism*.

4. Tibetan Writing adapted from Sanskrit. Ray, A. Reginald, *Indestructible Truth: The Living Spirituality of Tibetan Buddhism*, Shambhala, Boston & London 2012. Page 92.

5. Oral Tradition. *"Not committed to writing until several centuries after his death."* Lopez, Donald S. *"Buddha". Encyclopedia Britannica. https://www.britannica.com/biography/Buddha-founder-of-Buddhism*

6. Palm-leaf manuscript in Sanskrit. Pārameśvaratantra. Dated to the year 252, which some scholars judge to be of the era established by the Nepalese king Amśuvaran, therefore corresponding to 828 CE. Cambridge University Library MS Add.1049.1 – Wikipedia Commons Public Domain. Attribution: Ms Sarah Welch, CC BY-SA 4.0 <https://creativecommons.org/licenses/by-sa/4.0>, via Wikimedia Commons *https://commons.wikimedia.org/wiki/File:828_CE_Paramesvaratantra_Sanskrit_palm_leaf_manuscipt,_Late_Gupta_script,_Nepal.jpg*

7. Craig Lockard (2007.) *Societies, Networks, and Transitions*. Vol. I: *A Global History. "The Coming of Islam to India and Central Asia."* University of Wisconsin Press. p. 364. *ISBN 978-0-618-38612-3.*

8. Ray, A. Reginald, *Indestructible Truth: The Living Spirituality of Tibetan Buddhism*, Shambhala, Boston & London 2012. Page 78.

9. Ibid, page 102.

10. *Kværne, Per* (1995.) *The Bon Religion of Tibet: The Iconography of a Living Tradition*. Boston, Massachusetts: Shambhala. p. 13. ISBN 9781570621864.

11. "Tibetan Buddhism" - *Encyclopedia Britannica, https://www. britannica.com/topic/Tibetan-Buddhism.*

12. According to a commentary on the Vinaya Sutra known as 'Lung-Treng-Tik' in Tibetan by the First Dalai Lama (1392-1474), the Buddha is said to have emphasised several times the importance of pilgrimage. *https://www.buddhanet.net/e-learning/buddhistworld/ about-pilgrim.htm*

13. Sven Hedin, *Shigatse Dsong.* illustration from *Southern Tibet* by Sven Hedin (1917) Public domain, via Wikimedia Commons – Attribution: Sven Hedin, Public domain, via Wikimedia Commons. *https://commons.wikimedia.org/wiki/File:Sven_Hedin_Shigatse_ Dzong.jpg*

14. Circumambulation (Tibetan: Kora) - *https://tibetpedia.com/ lifestyle/kora-circumambulation/*

15. *https://buddhaweekly.com/wheel-dharma-prayer-wheels-may-ideal-buddhist-practice-busy-people-benefits-self-sentient-beings-teachers-say/*

16. Anapanasati Sutta (MN 118) – *dhammatalks.org*

17. Singh, Upinder. *A History of Ancient and Early Medieval India: From the Stone Age to the 12th Century.* Pearson. p. 25.

18. Bradley, Tamdin Sither (January 2001.) *"Tibetan Medicine - How and Why it Works"* the-south-asian.com   Retrieved 2023-05-17.

Chapter 3 - *The Way You Breathe Affects How You Feel And Live*

19. Anapanasati Sutta. *https://en.wikipedia.org/ wiki/%C4%80n%C4%81p%C4%81nasati_Sutta*

20. *"Ānāpānasati Sutra: Mindfulness of Breathing."* Majjhima Nikaya. Translated by Thanissaro Bhikkhu. dhammatalks.org. 2006. 118.

21. International Academy For Traditional Tibetan Medicine - *http:// www.iattm.net/uk/faculties/ttm-intro.htm*

22. Yin and Yang Symbol. Attribution: Klem, Public domain, Wikimedia Commons. *https://commons.wikimedia.org/wiki/ File:Yin_and_Yang_symbol.svg*

23. *Yin-Yang in Traditional Medicine and Its Relation to Parasympathetic (NO-cGMP) and Sympathetic (CO-cAMP) Balance,* Wan-Chung Hu* Division of Clinical Chinese Medicine, National Research Institute of Chinese Medicine, Ministry of Health and Welfare, Taipei, Taiwan – *https://www.nricm.edu.tw/var/file/0/1000/attach/73/ pta_2245_1378576_30566.pdf*

24. Rogers RS, Wang H, Durham TJ, Stefely JA, Owiti NA, Markhard AL, et al. (2023) *Hypoxia extends lifespan and neurological function in a mouse model of aging.* PLoS Biol 21(5): e3002117. *https://doi. org/10.1371/journal.pbio.3002117*

25. Schünemann HJ, Dorn J, Grant BJ, Winkelstein W Jr, Trevisan M. *Pulmonary function is a long-term predictor of mortality in the general population*: 29-year follow-up of the Buffalo Health Study. Chest. 2000 Sep;118(3):656-64. doi: 10.1378/chest.118.3.656. PMID: 10988186.

26. Michael Grant White, overview of Framingham Study on Longevity and Breathing. Published in Science News Vol.120. August 1, 1981. *https://optimalbreathing.com/pages/making-old-age-measure-up*

27. Vital Capacity - David S, Sharma S. *Vital Capacity.* [Updated 2023 Jul 24]. In: StatPearls [Internet]. Treasure Island (FL): StatPearls Publishing; 2024 Jan-. Available from: *https://www.ncbi.nlm.nih. gov/books/NBK541099/*

28. Harvard Medical School Health Newsletter – *Breathing Life Into Your Lungs*, April 2018. *https://www.health.harvard.edu/ newsletter_article/breathing-life-into-your-lungs*

29. Lewis A, Philip KEJ, Lound A, Cave P, Russell J, Hopkinson NS. *The physiology of singing and implications for 'Singing for Lung Health' as a therapy for individuals with chronic obstructive pulmonary disease.* BMJ Open Respir Res. 2021 Nov;8(1):e000996. doi: 10.1136/

bmjresp-2021-000996. PMID: 34764199; PMCID: PMC8587358. *https://www.ncbi.nlm.nih.gov/pmc/articles/PMC8587358/*

30. American Lung Association. *https://www.lung.org/lung-health-diseases/wellness/exercise-and-lung-health*

31. Normal Respiratory Rates. *https://www.medicalnewstoday.com/articles/324409#typical-rates*

32. *External rhythms can influence internal ones* – Dr Luciano Bernadi – *Circulation,* The Journal of the American Heart Association – European Perspectives in Cardiology – Dec 11, 2007. Extract: *https://www.ahajournals.org/doi/pdf/10.1161/circulationaha.107.187676*

33. British Medical Journal. *"Effect of rosary prayer and yoga mantras on autonomic cardiovascular rhythms"* comparative study - *https://www.bmj.com/content/323/7327/1446.full*

34. Bernardi L, Spadacini G, Bellwon J, Hajric R, Roskamm H, Frey AW. *Effect of breathing rate on oxygen saturation and exercise performance in chronic heart failure.* Lancet. 1998 May 2;351(9112):1308-11. do 10.1016/S0140-6736(97)10341-5. PMID: 9643792.

35. *Medical News Today. "What is a normal respiratory rate for your age."* Medically reviewed by Debra Sullivan, Ph.D., MSN, R.N., CNE, COI — By Adam Rowden — Updated on January 9, 2024 - *https://www.medicalnewstoday.com/articles/324409#atypical-rates*

Chapter 4 - *The Relationship Between Emotions & Breathing*

36. Philippot, P., Chapelle, G., & Blairy, S. (2002.) Respiratory feedback in the generation of emotion. Cognition and Emotion, 16(5), 605–627. *https://doi.org/10.1080/02699930143000392 - https://www.researchgate.net/publication/232965660_Respiratory_feedback_in_the_generation_of_emotion*

37. Folschweiller S, Sauer JF. *Respiration-Driven Brain Oscillations in Emotional Cognition.* Front Neural Circuits. 2021 Oct 27;15:761812. doi: 10.3389/fncir.2021.761812. PMID: 34790100; PMCID: PMC8592085.

Chapter 5 -*The Good and The Bad of Breathing*

38. *https://pubmed.ncbi.nlm.nih.gov/26335642/* - Guyenet PG, Bayliss DA. Neural Control of Breathing and CO_2 Homeostasis. Neuron. 2015 Sep 2;87(5):946-61. doi: 10.1016/j.neuron.2015.08.001. PMID: 26335642; PMCID: PMC4559867.

Chapter 6 - **Preparation For The T5T Breathing Exercises**

39. Olsson, Anders, *"Conscious Breathing"* Sorena AB; 3rd edition (August 1, 2014) page 62.

40. Endless Knot. Attribution: Don't panic (= Dogcow on de.Wikipedia), Public domain, via Wikimedia Commons – *https://commons. wikimedia.org/wiki/File:Endlessknot.svg*

41. *Recognizing and Treating Breathing Disorders* Edited by: Leon Chaitow, Dinah Bradley and Christopher Gilbert, page 146. *https://www.sciencedirect.com/topics/medicine-and-dentistry/ nasal-breathing*

42. Merck Manuals, *Control of Breathing, By Rebecca Dezube, MD, MHS, Johns Hopkins University https://www.msdmanuals.com/ home/lung-and-airway-disorders/biology-of-the-lungs-and-airways/ control-of-breathing*

43. Doctor A, Stamler JS. *Nitric oxide transport in blood: a third gas in the respiratory cycle.* Compr Physiol. 2011 Jan;1(1):541-68. doi: 10.1002/cphy.c090009. PMID: 23737185. *https://pubmed.ncbi. nlm.nih.gov/23737185/*

44. *Study Shows Blood Cells Need Nitric Oxide To Deliver Oxygen – https://www.medicalnewstoday.com/articles/292292*

45. *Why Do I Sometimes Get Stuffy In One Nostril? https://www. livescience.com/breathing-nose-sides* and *https://health. clevelandclinic.org/why-do-i-sometimes-get-stuffy-in-one-nostril*

46. Chaudhry R, Bordoni B. *Anatomy, Thorax, Lungs.* [Updated 2023 Jul 24]. In: StatPearls [Internet]. Treasure Island (FL): StatPearls Publishing; 2024 Jan-. Available from: *https://www.ncbi.nlm.nih. gov/books/NBK470197/*

47. Ochs, Matthias & Nyengaard, Jens & Jung, Anja & Knudsen, Lars & Voigt, Marion & Wahlers, Thorsten & Richter, Joachim &

Gundersen, Hans. (2004.) *The Number of Alveoli in the Human Lung.* American journal of respiratory and critical care medicine. 169. 120-4. 10.1164/rccm.200308-1107OC. *https://www.researchgate. net/publication/9078564_The_Number_of_Alveoli_in_the_Human_ Lung*

48. Ibid

Chapter 7 - *Experiencing Where The Breath Moves In Your Body*

49. *https://optimalbreathing.com/blogs/breathing-development-and-rehabilitation/breathing-exercises*

50. *https://optimalbreathing.com/blogs/emotional-issues/common-pitfalls-and-shortcomings-to-deep-breathing-exercises-techniques*

Chapter 8 - *How To Practice The Breathing Exercises With The Rites*

51. Residual Volume - LibreTexts Medicine. 22.3: The Process of Breathing - *https://med.libretexts.org/Bookshelves/Anatomy_and_ Physiology/Anatomy_and_Physiology_1e_(OpenStax)/Unit_5%3A_ Energy_Maintenance_and_Environmental_Exchange/22%3A_The_ Respiratory_System/22.03%3A_The_Process_of_Breathing*

52. Morton, A. R., K. King, S. Papalia, Carmel Goodman, K. R. Turley, and J. H. Wilmore. "Comparison of maximal oxygen consumption with oral and nasal breathing." *Australian journal of science and medicine in sport* 27, no. 3 (1995): 51-55. *https://pubmed.ncbi.nlm. nih.gov/8599744/*